Dr. Samuel V. Duh,
MD, MPH, FRSH

SAVING AFRICA FROM
HIV/AIDS
WE CAN DO IT

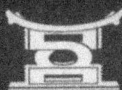

AFRAM PUBLICATIONS
(GHANA.) LIMITED.

Published by
Afram Publications (Ghana) Limited
P.O. Box M 18
Accra, Ghana.

First published 2008

ISBN 9964 70 426 7

Printed by

TABLE OF CONTENTS

Preface

PREFACE

On June 5, 1981 the United States Centers for Disease Control and Prevention (CDC) reported in their *Morbidity and Mortality Weekly Report (MMWR)* a mysterious disease that had killed five male homosexuals. Subsequent issues of the MMWR reported more cases of the mysterious disease in homosexuals. But in less than a year, the disease was being discovered among intravenous drug users, blood and blood product recipients, and, finally in heterosexuals. The victims all had one thing in common— previously healthy individuals with destroyed immune system. The disease was named *Acquired Immunodeficiency Syndrome (AIDS)*. Scientists quickly went to work to try to find the cause and cure for AIDS. They discovered the cause of the disease as a virus rather quickly and named it *Human Immunodeficiency Virus (HIV)*. It became quickly apparent that this disease was a worldwide problem, and soon it was recognized as a pandemic affecting almost every community worldwide.

As the pandemic widens and deepens, scientists continue their quest to find a way to halt it. But after more than 20 years of fighting the war on AIDS, we are nowhere near victory. Billions of dollars have been spent on the war. Major discoveries have been made in all spheres of research. Yet there is no cure; there is no vaccine; and educational efforts have not succeeded in preventing the spread of the disease to the degree it should have by now.

Devastating a disease as HIV/AIDS is, it is theoretically one hundred percent preventable. The fact that it is spreading out of control in many parts of the world is testimony to how society approaches problems. Human beings tend to want their problems to be solved quickly and to involve little or no personal sacrifice. So we demand that scientists come up with a cure for those already infected and a vaccine for those not infected. We often ignore important information regarding personal behaviour and continue to indulge in activities that put us at risk of acquiring the virus. Thus, we have taken the paradoxical approach to the pandemic by channelling more resources into "real" research to find a cure and vaccine than developing ways to effect individual responsibility for prevention.

Perhaps nowhere is the paradox of the HIV/AIDS pandemic more pervasive than in the continent of Africa. Most countries in Africa are among the least able to handle the devastation of HIV/AIDS, yet they are most affected by the pandemic. Africa, with only 10% of the world's population, had nearly 70% of people living with HIV/AIDS by the end of the year 2000. The epidemic has spread there faster than anywhere else in the world, and it has killed more people there than anywhere else. The purpose of this book is to discuss the HIV/AIDS situation in Africa and suggest some ways of dealing with it.

This book provides a comprehensive programmme to deal with all aspects of the epidemic in Africa. I believe that in order to control the epidemic, people must know the underlining causes of HIV/AIDS and how to deal with them. Therefore, in addition to the summary above, the first four chapters of the book deal with the general principles of history and epidemiology; transmission, pathogenesis, and clinical manifestations; and management of HIV disease. With that background, I then focus on the effect of the epidemic on Africa and how to deal with it.

The draft of the manuscript for this book was completed in 2001 when I lived in the United States. I moved to Ghana in July 2001 to take up a position with CARE International. Because of the process of moving and getting settled into a new job in a new environment, I did not have time to do the necessary polishing of the manuscript to be sent for publication. Therefore, some situations as discussed in the book might have changed by the time the book comes out. For example, by the end of 2000 (when the latest figures were available in 2001), the estimated number of people living with HIV/AIDS in the world was about 36 million; by the end of 2002 (the latest figure available in 2003 when the manuscript was being submitted for publication), the figure was 42 million; and when the book was going to press in 2006, the figure was 40 million (2005 figure).

I decided not to change the statistical information in relation to 2001 versus 2005 because firstly, by the time the book came out the figures would have changed again. Secondly, the magnitude of figure at the end of 2000 was so great that for discussion purposes and significance on the African continent, it doesn't really matter if we talk about 36 million or 40 million. More importantly, the issues of transmission, pathogenesis, clinical symptoms, and management remain the same. The important thing is the effect of the epidemic on the continent of Africa and how to deal with it. The effect of the HIV/AIDS epidemic on the continent of Africa is very dire indeed, but everything must be done to control it. And this book offers practical suggestion on controlling the epidemic in Africa. We can and must save Africa from the devastation of HIV/AIDS!

Though a lot of technical information is presented in this book, the language is simple enough that even clinical microbiology should be understood by the average reader. The book should be useful to doctors and other health care professionals, politicians and other policy makers, non-governmental organizations, private businesses, the clergy, and individuals who deal with all aspects of HIV/AIDS.

CHAPTER ONE

THE PARADOX OF THE AIDS EPIDEMIC

The title of this chapter is a phrase I coined in 1986, and the reasons for coining it still exist. The HIV/AIDS epidemic has been going on for more than 20 years, but not too much has changed in terms of society's reaction to it. Hence the paradox, which has existed since the time the acronym "AIDS" became a household word, persists.

The paradox of the HIV/AIDS epidemic consists of a triad of conflicting situations: 1. There appears to be too much information thrown at the public on the disease. 2. People tend to have unfounded fears about HIV/AIDS despite the (too much) information available to the contrary. 3. People continue to indulge in behaviours and activities, which put them at risk for the disease despite the information and the fear. These three conflicting situations existed in 1986 when I coined the phrase during a speech on HIV/AIDS, and they continue to exist today. Why?

Almost from the moment of identification of AIDS as a disease entity, popular and the scientific media have been saturated with information about it. Almost daily one reads something in the newspapers and magazines or hears something on the radio or television about HIV/AIDS. Almost every issue of scientific and medical journals carries an article or articles on HIV/AIDS. Several magazines and journals devoted entirely to the AIDS epidemic have come into existence. And in the current age of information technology, there are many websites that feature HIV/AIDS.

Hundreds of local and national AIDS conferences and symposia have taken place all over the world. And 13 international conferences had taken place in different countries through the summer of the year 2000. The World Health Organization, through its Global Programme on AIDS, convened an unprecedented meeting of ministers of health in January 1988 in London. Called the World Summit of Ministers of Health, the conference ended with a declaration on AIDS prevention with emphasis on broadening the scope of education and promoting exchange of information. In February 2000 the United Nations Security Council convened its first ever special session on a disease—HIV/AIDS. The vice president of the United States attended this unprecedented meeting in addition to top UN personnel and dignitaries, along with scientists from all over the world. And in June 2001, the UN General Assembly convened a special session on HIV/AIDS, the first ever General Assembly meeting devoted to a health issue that was attended by leaders from around the world. Also there have been several heads of state and government meetings in Africa to address the HIV/AIDS epidemic on that continent.

AIDS has been more studied in a relatively short time than any disease in history. More is known about the structure, molecular composition, behaviour, and target cells of the AIDS virus than any other virus in the world. The way the disease is spread was known even before the causative agent was identified. Indeed, there seems to be too much attention paid to and too much information about this one disease. Some people who have not been directly affected by the disease seem fed up with it. They are upset that so much attention has been and is being paid to AIDS, particularly with regard to resource allocation. What about other deadly or (more deadly) diseases?

Despite the appearance of too much information or information overkill, people still harbour a lot of unfounded fear about HIV/AIDS. The mention of AIDS in any setting manages to provoke all kinds of comments and reactions. Questions asked in 1981 about transmission from mosquitoes and other insects, through handshake with HIV/AIDS victims, from sweat and tears, and from donating blood are asked more than 20 years later. Fears about working in the same place with HIV/AIDS victims, children attending school with HIV/AIDS victims, and on the part of health care workers to treat HIV/AIDS patients still exist and persist. On one hand, we claim to have been educated to death about AIDS . . . too much information on HIV/AIDS; we don't need anymore. On the other hand, we are reluctant to accept the educational messages and continue to display unfounded fears. What a paradox!

The greatest paradox of all is the perpetuation of behaviours and activities that place us at risk for contracting HIV infection. The way the AIDS virus is transmitted has been clearly elucidated. Even before the virus was discovered, what to do or not to do to avoid getting the disease was known. Yet despite that knowledge and the profound fear people have of getting the disease, the activities that put us at risk persist, and in some situations seem to have been increasing. This is demonstrated by the fact that the disease continues to spread. Even more disturbing is the fact that communities which were spared the initial onslaught of the disease did not take advantage of the knowledge (and fear) to prevent the introduction of HIV/AIDS to those communities. Demographic groups that were not affected initially are now being affected in alarming proportions. The faces of AIDS have changed and continue to change. Not only are every demographic group and every community being affected, the rates of new HIV/AIDS cases are faster in the new groups than the "traditional" groups. At the same time, the rate has been decreasing among adult homosexuals. Yet the perception that AIDS is a homosexual disease still persists in some communities.

The success in slowing the rate of increase among homosexuals is largely due to the effective education in the homosexual community by members of that community. They took upon themselves to find out everything they possibly could about the disease in terms of education, research, and treatment programs. Those in the homosexual community with the means gathered the information and passed it on to others in the community. Hence the success in reducing the rates in that community while they continue to increase in other communities. Unfortunately, many young homosexuals have been ignoring the education available, and the disease is spreading fast among them. This phenomenon has largely resulted from the fact that new and powerful medications have helped prevent the quick death from AIDS, which was the norm before these medicines were discovered.

One of the biggest problems about the spread of HIV/AIDS has been its affecting teenagers. Since the average time from HIV infection to full-blown AIDS is about 10 years, infected teenagers develop AIDS when they are in their twenties. This is when they are in their most productive years of lives, and society is robbed of a substantial portion of its labour force. Paradoxically, younger people tend to live longer with AIDS and, therefore, exert longer drain on society's resources in addition to the loss of potential economic productivity.

Indeed, the vast majority of HIV/AIDS patients worldwide fall in the ages of 25 to 49. This age group is often the best-educated and most well trained workforce. Ordinarily, people in this age group are the healthiest since they are not old enough to acquire the most common crippling (age-related) diseases such as diabetes, heart disease, cancer, hypertension, and Alzheimer's. It is, therefore, a cruel irony that people in this productive age group should be affected to the degree that HIV/AIDS has.

Developing countries have particularly been dealt this devastating blow by nature. In the process of being transformed from mostly agrarian to industrialized nations, these countries rely on the technical expertise of their young people. Many of these countries had already been saddled with difficulties in controlling other diseases. Their economies had been weakened by wars, famine, and economic mismanagement. Therefore, with the HIV/AIDS epidemic, the very survival of some of them is at stake. In addition to losing a substantial portion of their workforce, the death of these young people leads to a mammoth orphan problem, adding to the economic hardship. Because of losing so many of their young people to HIV/AIDS, many countries in sub-Saharan Africa are struggling to survive.

The people who acquired AIDS in the early 1980s were largely infected before the AIDS virus and the means of transmission were identified. They had no choice in the matter in as much as they did not know their behaviour would result in a deadly disease. Many of those AIDS patients blamed themselves and were certainly blamed by some segments of society. Some of those who blamed themselves often stated that they would not have indulged in particular activities if they had known that those activities would lead to certain death. It stands to reason that armed with information on the activities which could lead to the acquisition of HIV/AIDS and the knowledge on how to avoid those activities, reasonable people would avoid them or at least take protective measures to minimize their chances of adverse outcome. If that had been the case, the AIDS epidemic would have reached a peak and started coming down. But that has certainly not been the case. The numbers of HIV/AIDS cases have been steadily going up throughout the world. Why?

As stated earlier, some countries and communities that were not affected initially have been reporting increasing numbers.

This should not have happened because of the availability of information. Similarly, the numbers continue to increase among teenagers despite availability of information. These are truly disturbing trends. Why did countries and communities not take the necessary measures to prevent HIV/AIDS from intruding them? And why do teenagers not take the necessary measures to avoid HIV/AIDS?

The two most common means of transmitting HIV are sexual intercourse and intravenous drug use (needle sharing). Individuals are reluctant to avoid these major activities. People do not want to avoid sexual intercourse entirely, and they are reluctant to employ the means of safer sex; that is, having sex with only one partner in a mutually exclusive relationship, and using condoms. Then there is the problem of prostitution. In some countries and communities, people, particularly young people, often engage in prostitution for economic survival. They concern themselves with daily economic survival than worrying about potential consequences of their behaviour. Intravenous drug users do not want to or cannot stop their habit because of addiction. Those who want to stop may not have access to drug treatment programs or clean needles. Some prostitutes are also drug users whose need for money is even greater because they need money for usual living and to support the drug habit.

It is disturbing that with the clear knowledge about the dangers involved with unprotected sexual activity and drug use, these practices are on the increase in many countries. These disturbing trends are likely due to denial. Countries and communities denied the fact that they needed to put in place effective preventive measures because they believed falsely that HIV/AIDS was the problem of certain countries and certain communities. They denied their people access to information or materials to promote prevention activities. They did not provide their people with the necessary means of prevention.

Some individuals, especially teenagers, deny that they could be infected with HIV, again because AIDS is someone else's disease. Also the feeling of invincibility among teenagers has contributed to the trend. So the activities that lead to increased risk of HIV infection such as homelessness, prostitution, drug use, multiple sexual partnerships are on the increase in this age group. Society seems to have missed the opportunity to prevent the introduction of HIV into a population group which was not born or old enough in 1981 when AIDS came to the scene. This group could have been totally protected from HIV infection had countries and communities put in place preventive measures when the means of transmission were first identified.

The war on AIDS has been fought amid controversy. There have been conflicting views among nations, within nations, within governments. There have been conflicts of government versus scientists; HIV/AIDS patients versus scientists; HIV/AIDS patients versus governments; scientists versus scientists. There has been hatred displayed against HIV/AIDS patients and so-called AIDS activists by some segments of society. On the other hand there have been alliances formed among different group and displays of compassion towards these patients. And HIV/AIDS patients in the homosexual community have received genuine affection from that community.

Some people have regarded AIDS as a divine curse; others have viewed it as an opportunity to express compassion. Some communities have objected to the presence of HIV/AIDS patients; others have embraced them. The HIV/AIDS epidemic has been regarded as a terrible burden on the health care system; it has been credited with permitting insights into other illnesses. The HIV/AIDS epidemic has brought about the institution of universal precautions in hospitals and other health care settings, making patient care safer for patient and health worker alike; yet the institution of universal precautions has added to the costs of health care. The AIDS epidemic has changed (for the better) the process by which new drugs and other technologies are approved. The term "differential pricing", by which drug companies sell the same drugs for different prices in different countries, came about because of the AIDS epidemic.

It is because of these and other paradoxes that the HIV/AIDS epidemic is in the current state of affairs. The causes and effects of these paradoxes need to be explored if the epidemic is to be controlled. After more than 20 years of fighting the war on AIDS we are nowhere near victory. Billions of dollars have been spent on the war. Major discoveries have been made in all spheres of research. Significant in this regard are the discovery of the causative agent, the development of blood tests to effect safe donated blood supply in many countries, and the development of therapeutic agents to increase the quality and quantity of life for HIV/AIDS patients. Yet there is no cure; there is no effective vaccine; and educational efforts have not succeeded in preventing the spread of the disease to the degree it should have by now. In the relatively short history of AIDS, there have been a lot of excitement and a lot of frustration.

Devastating a disease as HIV/AIDS is, it is theoretically one hundred percent preventable. The fact that it seems to be spreading out of control in many parts of the world is testimony to how society approaches problems. Human beings tend to want their problems solved quickly and to involve little or no personal sacrifice. We tend to want things done our way, to satisfy our individual needs. So we demand that scientists do something to discover a cure for those already infected and come up with a vaccine for those not infected. We do not want to take responsibility for our own behaviour. We often disregard important information when it comes to personal behaviour and assume that we are not going to be affected. Thus, we have taken a paradoxical approach to the epidemic by channelling more funds into "real" research to find a cure and vaccine than developing ways to effect individual responsibility for prevention.

There have been disagreements over whether and what to teach children about HIV/AIDS prevention. There has been controversy about whose job it is to teach about HIV/AIDS. There has been reluctance to implement programmes that might have a chance of protecting people from contracting HIV. Research has demonstrated that the use of condoms does help reduce the risk of transmission of sexually transmitted diseases, including HIV. Similarly, research has shown that the use of sterile needles by intravenous drug users does reduce the spread of HIV. Yet these means have been criticized as promoting sex and drug use.

Scientists also did not do an effective job in convincing the public about the need for individual responsibility in preventing HIV/AIDS during the first two decades of the epidemic. Indeed they seem to have contributed to the lack of interest in prevention activities on the part of the public. In addition to not actively focusing on prevention messages, scientists and the news media tended to play up on people's hopes about a cure. We often hear about the new discoveries and how close we are to finding a cure. Words like "breakthrough" have been used to describe steps towards finding a cure. The news media sometimes exaggerated such pronouncements. The public thus expects a cure or a vaccine soon and might not have seen a real need for individual responsibility, especially when such responsibility involves changes in habits that are strongly ingrained in us. Behaviour related to sex and drug use is supposed to be biologically based, socially sanctioned, and resistant to change (Fineberg, 1988).

Another confusing aspect of HIV/AIDS is how seemingly conflicting views are presented. On one hand, we hear that the AIDS virus is difficult to catch, and that we should not worry about catching it through casual contact. We almost have to want to get it before we can get it. In a speech in 1987, a former U.S. Surgeon General, C. Everret Koop, stated that most people did not have to worry about contracting AIDS. "Some people cannot get it even if they try," he said. On the other hand, we hear that it is easy to catch, and that everybody can get it. We are told everyone can get it, yet we hear of "risk groups", "risk behaviours", "risk areas". Some groups do not want to be stereotyped; yet they complain of not enough attention being paid to their particular (unique) situations. We are told to stay away from sex, alcohol and drugs, yet these activities are glamorised in the entertainment media.

Yes; the HIV/AIDS epidemic is full of paradoxes. We might be fighting a losing battle if we do not explore and deal with the paradoxes. There should be a reorientation of the approach to the HIV/AIDS epidemic. The focus should be on prevention, and effective ways should be explored to teach people about behaviour modification. This is important because as more is known about the AIDS virus, it has become clearer how difficult it is to come up with a cure. At the beginning of the epidemic, there seemed to be a commitment to focusing on preventive measures. When the virus was identified and more was learned about its structure and function, we lost the focus on prevention. Scientists and other policy makers channelled more resources to finding a cure and developing a vaccine.

Since 1986, I have been "preaching" that the focus on finding a cure and developing a vaccine is the wrong approach. The complexity of the AIDS virus makes such endeavours very difficult, if not impossible. I have often stated in my speeches that we should not "hold our breath" for a cure. No virus in history has been cured. Even the viruses that cause the common cold have eluded a cure after more than a hundred years of research. How do we expect a cure for such a complex virus as HIV if scientists have not been able to find a cure for cold viruses? I was, therefore, pleased by the focus on prevention at the 9th International Conference on AIDS in June 1993 in Berlin. The lack of progress on finding a cure, of coming up with an affective vaccine, and the uncertainty about the effectiveness of antiviral drugs in treating HIV infected people were boldly acknowledged. But alas, the prevention message was abandoned after the 11th International AIDS Conference in Vancouver in 1996.

It was at the Vancouver conference that the newly discovered antiretroviral medications called *protease inhibitors* were unveiled. Scientists actually talked about curing AIDS as paper after paper was presented on those medicines. For the first time, people with AIDS were living longer, healthier lives; some were even able to go back to work. Not only were they living longer, the new medicines were able to suppress the virus in their bodies to undetectable levels. And their CD4 cell count increased, all because of these new "miracle drugs". Once again, we abandoned the prevention message. People without AIDS started to indulge in activities and behaviours that put them at risk of acquiring the AIDS virus. The idea was if one got HIV infection from these behaviours, there were medicines to treat it. But yet again, we became disappointed. After a few years of phenomenal successes, problems with the protease inhibitors started cropping up. Scientists started sounding the caution note again. We were back to square one.

Perhaps nowhere is the paradox of the HIV/AIDS epidemic more pervasive than on the continent of Africa. Africa with 10% of the world's population had 70% of people living with HIV/AIDS by the end of the year 2000. The epidemic has spread there faster than anywhere else in the world, and it has killed more people there than anywhere else. Yet African countries are the least able to deal with such a mammoth epidemic. They were already saddled with the inability to control such infectious diseases as tuberculosis, malaria, and diarrhoeal diseases before the AIDS epidemic hit the continent in the early 1980s. The problem with wars, famine, and economic mismanagement mentioned earlier are more evident in Africa than anywhere else.

The approach to the control of the epidemic in Africa is not unlike that in other parts of the world. There have been denial, complacency, and mismanagement. There has been lack of prevention effort by governments and institutions; and individual responsibility for their behaviour has been lacking just as it has been in other parts of the world. Yet virtually no country in Africa can afford the antiretroviral medications . . . if they continued to be effect. Paradoxically, African governments, activists, and other international organizations have been pleading, even demanding, that the drug companies make these drugs available and affordable in Africa. Meanwhile, people continue to indulge in activities that put them at risk for the disease.

The lack of progress in finding a cure for AIDS, of coming up with an effective vaccine, and the lack of research on effective prevention measures go on as the epidemic rages on. Opportunities have been missed on the prevention front as more effort has been focused on "real science" to find a cure and vaccine. Meanwhile "Africa is burning". How long can the "burning" go on? How is the "fire" going to be put out? Who is going to put out the fire? These are difficult questions but they must be answered and answered quickly before a whole continent is damaged beyond repair. It is totally unacceptable to declare Africa a lost continent because of HIV/AIDS. We can save Africa from HIV/AIDS.

REFERENCES

1. Cimons, M (1991, June 2). Disease has brought society's best and worst. *Daytona Beach News Journal* 1, p. 4A

2. Duh, S.V. (1991). *Blacks and AIDS: Causes and Origins,* Newbury Park: Sage Publications.

3. Fineberg, H.V. (1988). The social dimension of AIDS. *Scientific American,* 259, 128-134.

4. Thomas, L (1988). AIDS: An unknown distance still to go. *Scientific American,* 259, 152.

CHAPTER TWO

HISTORY AND EPIDEMIOLOGY OF HIV/AIDS

Acquired Immunodeficiency Syndrome was "born" in June 1981. In its weekly newsletter, *Morbidity and Mortality Weekly Report* (MMWR), the U.S. Centers for Disease Control and Prevention (CDC) introduced the world to a new disease. An issue of MMWR in June 1981 discussed *Pneumocystic carinii Pneumonia* (PCP) in five male homosexuals from Los Angeles. In another issue the next month, 26 cases of *Kaposi's sarcoma* in male homosexuals from New York were discussed. The CDC then warned physicians to be alert for PCP, Kaposi's sarcoma, and other "opportunistic infections" in homosexual men (CDC, 1981).

The CDC had often warned physicians (and the public) to look out for the unusual occurrence of certain diseases. Such warnings were usually on existing diseases with unusual occurrence, such as outbreaks of Cholera or Salmonella. However, the warning about PCP and Kaposi's sarcoma was of a different type. The patients with those illnesses that prompted the warning had two things in common—they were all male homosexuals, and they all had immune system suppression. The warning, thus, referred to opportunistic infections associated with immuno-suppression *in homosexual men*. Furthermore, the disease did not respond to the usual therapy, and the patients all died. Little did anyone know at that time that those few cases would lead to an epidemic, indeed a pandemic. .

The doctors who saw these patients and the CDC scientists were puzzled at the beginning. Both PCP and Kaposi's sarcoma were unusual in that they had not occurred in previously healthy young individuals. PCP had occurred in individuals whose immune system was failing, such as people on chemotherapy or with kidney disease; and Kaposi's sarcoma occurred in elderly men also with weakened immune system. Why were they occurring in previously healthy men? And why did the men have immune suppression? It became obvious quickly that a new disease, at that time restricted to homosexuals, was at hand. Some clinicians referred to it as *gay (homosexual) immuno-suppression disease*. A search was mounted to find more cases of this unusual condition and find out what was causing it.

It became evident rather quickly that the new disease was not just a homosexual disease. In less than a year, people outside the homosexual community were demonstrating the same symptoms. Scientists became even more puzzled. When the disease seemed to be restricted to homosexuals, there was the logical speculation that there was something in homosexual men or their sexual behaviour that led to the immune system suppression. But when people outside the homosexual community started falling to the disease, the mystery surrounding the disease became even more glaring. The search for the cause of the new disease became more urgent. Some people in the homosexual community asserted that the urgency with which scientists were approaching the search was predicated on the fact that the condition was spreading beyond the homosexual community.

The new disease quickly captured the attention of scientists, politicians, and the general public alike. It quickly evolved from an obscure "homosexual" disease to a pandemic affecting all segments of society. It captured the curiosity of the scientific world, and an unprecedented race was mounted to search for its cause. The breakneck speed initiated at the beginning has continued through the years in an attempt to control the epidemic. This mammoth effort has been rewarded with a tremendous amount of information and knowledge about the disease. Yet there is no cure or vaccine for the disease, and educational efforts to prevent it have not yielded the required results. There is no doubt that more needs to be done . . . by everyone (not just governments and scientists) to control the pandemic.

History

As scientists were struggling to identify a cause for the new disease, it became quickly apparent that it was not just a homosexual disease. By early 1982, it had been found among intravenous drug users, and later in July that year among hemophiliacs. Then it was found in recipients of blood transfusion, heterosexuals, and infants in the United States and Europe in early 1983. Later that year, it was found among Haitians and people in central Africa, neither group with significant history of homosexuality or drug use. By 1985, it was being found in many other countries on every continent. In 1986, the World Health Organization (WHO) initiated a programme, WHO Special Programme on AIDS, to deal with the worldwide AIDS problem. It had become a true pandemic. Later WHO changed the name of the special programme to the Global Programme on AIDS to reflect the pandemic nature of the disease. In 1996 the WHO programme became integrated with other United Nations agencies to form the Joint United Nations Programme on HIV/AIDS (UNAIDS).

The work on the new disease was multi-facetted. As some scientists searched for the cause of the disease, others worked on establishing the means of transmission, how the disease was passed from person to person, and why it was causing the patients to die. First, it was established that something was causing the victims' immune system to break down. Then the means of transmission became fairly clear. It became evident that the disease was transmitted sexually, and the most important indicator was the number of sexual partners, not necessarily the sexual preference. Then it was postulated that blood might be involved in the transmission somehow because of the prevalence in IV drug users, blood transfusion recipients, and hemophiliacs. Thus, it was suggested that the cause might be an infectious agent, based on the means of transmission. Some scientists suggested a single infectious agent, while others postulated a combination of agents.

By 1982, a case-definition had been established for reporting purposes. That is, individuals displaying a set of symptoms were to be diagnosed as having the disease, and doctors seeing them should report the cases to the CDC. (The case-definition was revised in 1987 and again in 1992). The collection of symptoms common to the patients of the disease was unique, and scientists concluded that they were dealing with an entirely new disease. They named it *Acquired Immunodeficiency Syndrome*. Its acronym AIDS quickly became a household word, as AIDS was being diagnosed in all corners of the globe.

The postulation of means of transmission was the most important discovery in the early part of the epidemic. This is because that discovery enabled the U.S. Public Health Service to issue recommendations for AIDS prevention in early 1983, almost a full year before the causative agent was discovered (Heyward & Curran, 1988). Remarkably, more than 20 years later, those recommendations are valid today and serve as the backbone of HIV/AIDS prevention activities. The discovery of the causative agent came in record time. A single virus was identified in January 1984 as the causative agent of AIDS.

The underlying defect for the development of AIDS was the destruction of the immune system, specifically the depletion of the immune cells called *T4 cells*. Possible causes of the T4 cell destruction considered were bacteria, viruses, fungi, or even non-infectious agents such as the drug *amylnitrite* and over-exposure to sperm. Regarding sperm, it was first thought that perhaps repeated exposure to sperm during homosexual intercourse caused the T4 cell destruction. However, when AIDS started to be found in other population groups, scientists started looking for other possible causes.

Teams of scientists in the United States and France simultaneously focused on the likelihood of a virus as the causative agent. They based their search on two pieces of evidence: It had already been established that a retrovirus called *Human T-cell lymphotrophic virus I* (HTLV-I) could be transmitted sexually and by blood; and a retrovirus of cats called *Feline Leukaemia Virus* (FeLV) could cause cancer and immune system suppression (Gallo & Montagnier, 1988). Putting the two pieces of information together, they hypothesized that AIDS could be caused by a retrovirus that was transmitted by sexual intercourse and by blood, and that virus caused T4 cell destruction.

The French team first isolated a retrovirus from lymph nodes of homosexual men with AIDS. Later, the U.S. team isolated the same virus from homosexual AIDS patients. Further work led to the isolation of a single retrovirus from several AIDS patients in several countries in January 1984. That retrovirus was declared the causative agent of AIDS. The French team, led by Dr. Luc Montagnier of the Pasteur Institute, named the new virus *Lymphadenopathy-Associated Virus* (LAV). The U.S. team, headed by Dr. Robert Gallo of the National Cancer Institute, named it *Human T-cell Lymphotrophic Virus III* (HTLV-III). The virus then became officially known as HTLV-III/LAV to satisfy both teams of scientists. Much later the virus was renamed *Human Immunodeficiency Virus* (HIV).

The next major accomplishment by scientists was the detection of antibodies to the virus soon after it was isolated. Antibodies to the virus were found in both patients with AIDS and in non-patients. The detection of antibodies in individuals without AIDS led to more understanding of the disease process. It became evident quickly that AIDS was the end stage of the disease, and that an asymptomatic state existed during which people infected with the virus could be perfectly healthy. Furthermore, those with asymptomatic infection could transmit the virus to others.

The discoveries of HIV and antibodies to the virus were two giant steps in AIDS research. They gave the hope for eventual, perhaps quick, control of the epidemic. If the virus that causes the disease and means of detecting it were known, then the development of a cure would be easy. Also, scientists would (quickly) come up with a vaccine since a single causative agent had been identified, and it could be tested for. However, more than 20 years after the identification of the virus, there is no cure; there is no vaccine; and the transmission of the virus continues virtually uninhibited.

But it has not all been bad news. In 1985, laboratory tests were licensed for the detection of antibodies to HIV. The tests have been used both for screening and diagnostic purposes. The *enzyme-linked immunosorbent assay* (ELISA) technique is a serologic or test tube test, and it is used for quick screening. The Western Blot (WB), the more elaborate electrophoresis technique, is used to confirm a positive ELISA test. Since June 1985, all donated blood for transfusion has been tested for HIV antibodies in many countries. All blood testing positive or indeterminate for HIV antibodies is discarded. This has virtually eliminated transfusion-associated transmission of HIV in most countries, a no mean fete indeed. However, like all laboratory tests, those for

HIV antibodies are not 100% accurate; there is a very small chance that blood that has tested negative for HIV antibodies could be infected with HIV. It has been estimated that about 1 in 225,000 chance exists for acquiring HIV infection through donated blood. But in some less developed countries screening blood for HIV is not as effective as it is in more advanced countries, and there is a higher chance of HIV transmission through blood transfusion.

There are two potential problems with screening donated blood for HIV even under the best of laboratory conditions. The first is false negative results. Though the tests are 99% sensitive and 99% specific (sensitivity means a positive test result is truly positive, and specificity means a negative result is truly negative), a blood sample could actually carry HIV and still test negative. The second phenomenon has to do with how long the donor has been infected with HIV. There is a so-called "window period" during which an infected person has not yet built up enough antibodies to the virus to show up as a positive test. The window period ranges from about two weeks to about six months after infection. Despite these two potential errors in laboratory tests for HIV antibodies, blood supply is quite safe, at least in developed countries.

After HIV was isolated, the next task was to study its structure and function in order to find ways of destroying it. The virus has been thoroughly studied, its chemical structure has been well elucidated, and where it attaches itself on human cells is well known. It is a retrovirus that uses the genetic material of human cells to reproduce itself. The simplest way to cure HIV infection is to prevent the virus from reproducing itself, in effect, to kill the virus dead in its tracks. But this has not been easy to accomplish, though several drugs have been developed to do just that.

The first anti-AIDS drug, really anti-HIV drug, *Azidothymidine* (AZT) or *Retrovir* was approved for use in 1987. It works by inhibiting an enzyme called *reverse transcriptase* that is required by the virus in the process of producing itself. Most AIDS patients taking AZT felt better and lived longer, but the medicine has severe side effects, and it has been unable to effect a cure. Beside the side effects, it was taken 200 mg five times a day, often requiring the patient to set an alarm clock to wake up in the middle of the night to take the medicine. Other anti-HIV drugs have been developed, and both *Didanosine* (ddI) and *Dideoxycytosine* (ddC) were approved in 1992. They both work similarly to AZT by inhibiting reverse transcriptase. They had fewer side effects than AZT but their two major side effects—pancreatitis and severe peripheral neuropathy—were more incapacitating.

The first three drugs approved for the treatment of AIDS belonged to a group called *Nucleoside Reverse Transcriptase Inhibitors* (NRTIs). The indication for use of ddI and ddC is for patients who had failed to respond to AZT or had been unable to tolerate it. Also, both have been used in combination with AZT. The idea behind combination therapy is that smaller doses of two or more medicines would work together to produce more antiviral effect without the severe side effect each high dose causes. Also the combination makes it less likely for HIV to become resistant to the drug.

AZT has been the most widely used antiretroviral agent of AIDS, indeed for the spectrum of HIV infection. In 1990, a research group in the United States called the AIDS Clinical Trial Group (ACTG) in its Protocol 019 demonstrated that AZT was effective at lower doses than what had been used to treat AIDS since 1987. With that discovery it was recommended that 500 mg of AZT a day be used to treat individuals with HIV infection who had not yet developed AIDS. However, because it was still quite toxic even at that lower dose, it should be given to only those whose T4 cell count was below 500 cells/ml. The U.S. Food and Drug Administration (FDA) subsequently approved the use of AZT to treat asymptomatic HIV infection. In June 1993, researchers published preliminary results of a long term study in England and France which showed that AZT was not effective in slowing the progression of HIV infection to AIDS when used over long periods of time (Aboulker & Swart, 1993). Furthermore HIV started developing resistance to all three NRTIs.

Absent an effective drug to kill the virus, other approaches have been tried and are being researched to treat AIDS patients. These have included immuno-modulators, chemicals that boost the body's immune system, and bone marrow transplantation. Some so-called alternative medicines such as Compound Q from the Chinese periwinkle plant and various other herbal medicines have also been tried. Heat therapy, during which a patient's blood was superheated, supposedly to kill all HIV, and put back into the patient, had a rather short life. A few patients died after undergoing heat therapy, so it quickly went out of favour. In addition, reports of new "breakthrough" medicines to cure AIDS are often given by the news media. In this regard it was announced in July 1993 that Thalidomide, the anti-miscarriage medicine that caused thousands of deformed infants in the 1960s, had shown promise in curing the AIDS virus. Meanwhile, various therapeutic modalities are employed to treat the many opportunistic diseases that define AIDS with varying degrees of success.

Because of the fact that none of the NRTIs could effect a cure for AIDS, and because of their numerous problems with side effects and resistance, research went on to discover other antiretroviral medications. A group of medications that also inhibit the reverse transcriptase enzyme was discovered. This particular group belongs to a class called *Non-nucleoside Reverse Transcriptase Inhibitors* (NNRTIs). The NNRTIs were to be used in combination with or instead of the NRTIs. Like their NRTIs predecessors, the NNRTIs have bad side effects, and the virus quickly developed resistance to these new drugs. But the true revolution in the management of HIV/AIDS came with the discovery of a new class called *Protease Inhibitors* (PIs).

The PIs work at a different level of the reproductive cycle of the virus from the NRTIs and NNRTIs. When they went into routine use in 1996, people started talking about a cure for AIDS. In combination with the other classes or alone, patients taking PIs felt much better, lived longer, and had their viral load drop and T4 cell count go up. And death rates from AIDS declined in countries where the protease inhibitors were available. For example, in the United States, death rates declined by 42% between 1996 and 1997 and by 20% between 1997 and 1998. Again the PIs had side effects, and their use involved the taking of many pills at different times by the patient. But after a few years of use, the virus once again developed resistance to the PIs. Furthermore, the use of PIs and the other classes of medication are very expensive indeed, and they have been out of reach to many HIV/AIDS patients in both the developed and developing countries. By the end of the year 2000, 16 different medications belonging to the three classes of drugs were in general use. Research goes on to find other drugs to get around the problems attendant to the current drugs.

The second approach to the control of HIV is the use of vaccines. The projected use of vaccination in AIDS is both therapeutic and preventive. In terms of therapeutic vaccinations, the vaccine would be given to patients who already have AIDS or HIV infection. The vaccine would theoretically neutralize HIV and thereby halt the relentless destruction of T4 cells so that HIV infected people would not go on to develop AIDS, and AIDS patients might recover. Preventive vaccine would be given to people who have not yet been exposed to HIV so that if and when exposure occurred, they would not develop HIV infection and AIDS. The latter approach is akin to standard vaccination for measles, polio, and the like.

Like the search for a cure, the search for a vaccine has been going on since HIV was identified. Researchers in different parts of the world have been working on different aspects of vaccine development, but there is still no vaccine available for AIDS control. Two major obstacles have complicated the work on vaccine:

1. There are several strains of HIV, making it difficult to find a

vaccine that can control all the many strains. 2. The second problem has to do with the fact that the virus is so dangerous. The most effective vaccines are those made from the whole virus. But the virus is so dangerous that few scientists are willing to discuss the whole virus vaccine for HIV. Most scientists have been trying to isolate a protein from the virus that would be potent enough to stimulate immune response in humans but weak enough not to cause HIV infection. A lot of work has gone on and is going on in various laboratories all over the world on vaccine development using this approach. Meanwhile, some people have suggested that drug companies and other manufacturers have been dragging their feet regarding coming up with an AIDS vaccine because of fears of liability.

The problem of multiple strains of HIV is a particularly vexing one. The development of a vaccine for an organism is complicated if the organism has several strains, but it can be done as it is the case with the influenza virus. However, unlike influenza, HIV is a new virus that seems to be evolving. The distinct forms of HIV are believed to result from mutation of the virus, and the fact that so many strains have been discovered in such a short time indicates that HIV is mutating quite rapidly (Steinberg, 1992). Therefore, not only is it difficult to develop a multiple-strain vaccine but new strains might have appeared by the time such a vaccine is put into routine use because of the fast rate of mutation.

In addition to the multiple strains of HIV, there are distinct retroviruses causing AIDS or AIDS-like illness. The first of these is HIV-2 isolated in 1985 from prostitutes and surgical patients in Senegal. Since then the common AIDS virus was referred to as HIV-1 in scientific circles. Subsequently, HIV-2 was isolated from people with AIDS-like illness in several other West African countries, Portugal, and several other European countries. HIV-2 was first isolated in the United States in 1988 from a patient who emigrated from West Africa and had developed the AIDS-like illness in his home country before going to the U.S. In July 1988, Dr. Guido Vander Groen of the Institute of Tropical Medicine in Antwerp, Belgium, isolated yet another retrovirus from a man and his wife in Cameroon, West Africa. That virus was named HIV-3. However, HIV-2 is the most common of the other retroviruses. HIV-2 is immunologically different from HIV-1 but both viruses appear to be transmitted through sexual contact and contaminated blood. However, HIV-2 infection progresses more slowly to AIDS and causes less severe symptoms. It is found mostly in West African countries, but many cases have been found in other parts of the world. This prompted the U.S. Food and Drug Administration in 1993 to mandate the testing of all donated blood for HIV-2 in addition to HIV-1. After the initial fears of HIV-2 subsided, that particular type of retrovirus did not seem to have taken hold, as has HIV-1. So by the early 1990s, HIV-2 had virtually disappeared from the AIDS lexicon; so when scientists now refer to HIV, they are talking about HIV-1.

As the search for an effective vaccine went on and it was complicated by the fact that there were so many different strains, many scientists worked in different laboratories around the world to overcome that problem. In 1996, the International AIDS Vaccine Initiative (IAVI) was formed to allow scientists to share ideas and support each other's efforts. Also, as an organization, IAVI is more able to raise funds than individual scientists can. It has been working diligently since, but there is no usable vaccine. At the XIII International AIDS Conference in Durban, South Africa, in July 2000, IAVI announced several initiatives with the hope of having a usable vaccine in the next five to ten years.

An uncommon complication of the control effort is the contention by some researchers that AIDS is not caused by HIV alone or not at all. There has been a debate for years that something(s) works in combination with HIV to produce the immune system destruction in AIDS patients—the so-called cofactor theory. Dr. Luc Montagnier, the co-discoverer of HIV, has espoused this theory. He has suggested that a microorganism called *Mycoplasma*, which is not a virus, is the co-factor organism. Some other scientists have suggested that HIV is not the causative agent of AIDS.

The final approach to the control of the HIV/AIDS pandemic is prevention education to effect individual behaviour modification. As stated in Chapter One, this disease is potentially 100% preventable. Even before HIV was identified as the causative agent, the means of transmission were rather clear. Modifying certain human behaviours would prevent the transmission. Except for blood transfusion, the other means involve what we as human beings do or not do to protect ourselves. With the screening of donated blood, almost all new infections have been through illicit drug use (needle sharing) and sexual activity. But people do not want to or cannot abstain from these activities.

Drug users are addicted to the particular drugs they use and cannot easily walk away from them. However, governments and institutions have been reluctant to provide treatment facilities for those who want to use them. They have also been unwilling to provide users with clean needles for fear of encouraging drug use. Sex is supposed to be biologically based, socially sanctioned, and resistant to change (Feinberg, 1988). So as the rates of HIV/AIDS continue to increase, activities such as prostitution, multiple sexual partnership, and casual sex go on all over the world. Most people do not want to abstain from sex, and many do not want to use or cannot afford condoms.

There is no doubt that preventive education works, but not enough emphasis has been placed on prevention. When modest gains were made in the United States in this regard, those efforts were slowed or stopped when the protease inhibitors became available to treat HIV/AIDS patients. Some individuals who might otherwise have taken precautions decided to take risks and hope they would not contract HIV infection; and if they did, there were effective medications to treat them. There have been some significant successes in some countries when education has been taken seriously. Countries like Thailand, Uganda, and Senegal have been able to reduce their rates of HIV/AIDS through aggressive educational campaigns and making condoms available free of charge or at low costs. But most other countries have not emulated the examples of these countries, and the pandemic rages on with virtually every country on earth being affected.

Epidemiology

The discovery of AIDS as a disease entity and as an epidemic was mainly through the work of scientists called *Epidemiologists*.

These specialists study the occurrence and distribution of diseases and their control in populations. Often called medical detectives, epidemiologists use surveillance information to arrive at determinants of diseases, much the way criminal detectives use such information to unravel the mysteries of crimes. In this process, epidemiologists at the CDC came upon some intriguing surveillance information in June, 1981. They received a report of five cases of an extremely rare type of pneumonia called *Pneumocystis carinii pneumonia* (PCP) all occurring within the previous eight months. The CDC had received only two case reports of PCP between November 1967 and December 1979. A month later, surveillance information on another rare illness, *Kaposi's sarcoma*, reached the CDC. That cancer had very rarely been seen in the U.S. and had occurred only in older men; yet the 26 cases had occurred within the previous 30 months in young men (Heyward & Curran, 1988).

An epidemic is defined as the occurrence of a disease at a rate higher than expected. Therefore, though the numbers of PCP and Kaposi's sarcoma were relatively small, the epidemiologists knew that they were dealing with an epidemic. However, they had no idea that it was going to be such a massive epidemic. Dr. James Curran, who headed the team of epidemiologists at CDC that investigated the first reported cases, is quoted as saying: "I remember people coming to my office in 1981 and saying, 'if the trends keep on going this way, we could have 1,000 cases of this disease'. I said, that's being pessimistic. I hope it never gets that bad." (Cimons, 1991; p. 4A). Obviously, Dr. Curran's hope has been shattered by multiples of factors. The UNAIDS estimated that 36.1 million people world were living with HIV/AIDS by the end of the year 2000, a huge jump from Dr. Curran's fear of 1,000.

The distribution of AIDS cases in the world was uneven during the early part of the epidemic. It was also unevenly distributed within countries. This prompted the World Health Organization (WHO) to recognize three patterns of geographic distribution:

Pattern 1.

Most cases of AIDS occur in homosexual/bisexual men and IV drug users. Heterosexual transmission is responsible for a relatively few cases, although the rate of heterosexual transmission is increasing. Consequently, the majority of AIDS cases are men. The overall national infection rate is probably less than 1% with certain segments of the population having in excess of 50%. The United States, most European countries, and some Latin American countries appear to follow this pattern.

Pattern 2.

Most cases occur in heterosexuals. Transmission through homosexual/bisexual activity and IV drug use is rare. Consequently, male to female ratio of AIDS cases approximates 1. The overall national infection rate is probably more than 1% and may exceed 15% in sexually active young adult populations of some urban areas. Most African countries and several Latin American countries appear to follow this pattern.

Pattern 3.

HIV has only recently been introduced to these countries. The majority of cases originated outside the country. No homosexual/ IV drug use or heterosexual transmission pattern has emerged. The majority of Asian countries, countries in North Africa and most countries in Oceania follow this pattern (WHO Special Programme on AIDS, 1987).

In an earlier book (Duh, 1991), I criticized this WHO distribution pattern because it seemed to reinforce the notion that HIV is transmitted differently in different population groups or by unique individual characteristics. As will be discussed in the next chapter, HIV transmission requires exposure of the virus to blood contact irrespective of the population group. Furthermore, people in Pattern 3 areas might falsely believe that they were not at risk for AIDS. Indeed, this has been borne out. Governments and individuals in those countries did not take the necessary steps to prevent AIDS from taking hold in their countries. Consequently, many more cases of AIDS are being reported from those areas of the world; and HIV infection is spreading very fast there, with alarming rates in India, Thailand, some parts of China, and some of the former Soviet republics. As late as August, 1990 five countries had reported a total of only 107 cases from Southeast Asia to WHO; just 10 years later, UNAIDS estimated HIV/AIDS cases in this region at 5.8 million at the end of 2000!

The AIDS epidemic has long been a pandemic; that is, it is present in all corners of the world, and almost every country is being affected. Table 2.1 demonstrates the global summary of the pandemic as of the end of the year 2000. From the beginning of the epidemic, it was unevenly distributed in the world and within countries. Table 2.2 demonstrates the uneven distribution by region and by gender, with sub-Saharan Africa bearing the brunt of the pandemic. It was also unevenly distributed among demographic groups within countries. However, the demographics have been changing. For example, in 1981, fully 97% of AIDS cases in the United States were in males with about 79% being in male homosexuals; in 2000, 20% of estimated cases were females. A similar situation existed in Africa where the ratio of male to female was close to 1, with a slight edge for males in the early to mid-1980s; by 2000, 55% of estimated cases were females.

The control of the pandemic, whether with medications, vaccines, or behaviour modification would have to take into consideration the epidemiology of the pandemic. The uneven distribution requires an understanding of the transmission of HIV and disease process of AIDS and how that process affects different populations. By so doing, more meaningful approaches could be designed to control the epidemic at different settings, taking the epidemiology of HIV/AIDS into consideration.

Table 2. I.   GLOBAL SUMMARY OF THE HIV/AIDS
EPIDEMIC, DECEMBER 2000

Number of people living with HIV/AIDS

Total	**36.1 million**
Adults	34.7 million
Women	16.4 million
Children < 15	1.4 million

Total number of deaths since the beginning of epidemic: **21.8 million**

Adults	17.5 million
Women	9 million
Children < 15	4.3 million

Number of people newly infected in 2000

Total	**5.3 million**
Adults	4.7 million
Women	2.2 million
Children	600,000

AIDS death in 2000

Total	**3 million**
Adult	2.1 million
Women	1.3 million
Children <15	500,000

SOURCE: Joint United Nations Programme on HIV/AIDS (UNAIDS)

Table 2.2.   GLOBAL SUMMARY OF HIV/AIDS BY REGION, END
OF 2000

Region	Adults & Children Living with HIV/AIDS	Adult Prevalence	% of HIV Positive Adults who are Women
Sub-Saharan Africa	25.3 million	8.8%	55%
North Africa & Middle-East	400,000	0.20	40%
South & South-East Asia	5.3 million	0.56%	35%
East Asia & Pacific	640,000	0.07%	13%
Latin America	1.4 million	0.50%	25%
Caribbean	390,000	2.3%	35%
Eastern Europe & Central Asia	700,000	0.35%	25%
Western Europe	540,000	0.24%	25%
North America	920,000	0.6%	20%
Australia & New Zealand	15,000	0.13%	10%
Total	**36.1 million**	**1.1%**	**47%**

SOURCE: Joint United Nations Programme on HIV/AIDS (UNAIDS)

REFERENCES

1. Aboulker, J. & Swart A. (1993). Preliminary analysis of the Concorde trial. *Lancet*, 889-890.
2. American Health Consultants (1993). Benefits of alpha interferon will be put to clinical test. *AIDS Alert*, 8, 58-60
3. Are you prepared for HIV-2? *Emergency Medicine*,1993, 25, 109-110.
4. Centers for Disease Control (1981). *Pneumocystis* pneumonia: Los Angeles. *MMWR*, 30, 250-252.
5. Centers for Disease Control (1991). The HIV/AIDS epidemic: The first 10 years. *MMWR*, 40, 357.
6. Centers for Disease Control (1993). Impact of the expanding AIDS case definition on AIDS reporting—United States, first quarter, 1993. *MMWR*, 42, 308-310.
7. Cimons. M. (1991, June 2). Disease has brought society's best and worst. *Daytona Beach News Journal*, p. 4A.
8. Duh, S.V. (1991). *Blacks and AIDS: Causes and Origins*, Newbury Park: Sage Publications.
9. Ellerbrock, T.V., et al (1991). Epidemiology of women with AIDS in the United States, 1981 through 1990. *Journal of American Medical Association*, 265, 2971-2975.
10. Fauci, A. S. (1993). CD4+ T-lymphocytopenia without HIV infection no lights, no camera, just facts. *New England Journal of Medicine*, 328, 429-430.
11. Gallo, R.C. & Montagnier, L. (1988). AIDS in 1988. *Scientific American*, 259, 40-51.
12. Global STD picture grim and worsening. *STD Bulletin*, 1992, 11, 3.
13. Heyward, W.L. & Curran, J.W. (1988). The epidemiology of AIDS in the U.S. *Scientific American*, 259, 72-81.
14. Ho, D.D., et al (1993). Idiopathic CD4+ T- lymphocytopenia immunodeficiency without evidence of HIV infection. *New England Journal Medicine*, 328, 380-385.
15. Levi, J & Kates, J. (2000) HIV: challenging the health care delivery system. *American Journal of Public Health,* 90: 1033-1036.
16. Mann, J.M., et al (1988). The international epidemiology of AIDS.

Scientific American, 259, 82-89.

17. Marlink, R.G. & Essex, M. (1987). Africa and the biology of HIV infection. *Journal of American Medical Association,* 257, 2632-2633.

18. Smith, D.K., et al (1993). Unexplained opportunistic infections and CD4+ T lymphocytopenia without HIV infection. *New England Journal of Medicine,* 28, 374-379.

19. Steinberg, S. (1992). HIV comes in five family groups. *Science,* 256, 966.

CHAPTER THREE

TRANSMISSION OF HIV, AND PATHOGENESIS AND CLINICAL MANIFESTATIONS OF AIDS

As stated in Chapter One, AIDS has been more studied and more information has been disseminated about it in a relatively short period of time than any other disease in history. However, there appears to be a rather widespread lack of adequate knowledge about the condition. Since 1986, I have been giving presentations on HIV/AIDS to various groups including doctors, other hospital and health care employees, news media personnel, and the general public. I have also served as a consultant to businesses, hospital boards, and school boards on the development of work place HIV/AIDS policy. In all these encounters, I have often been asked questions by doctors and lay people alike that demonstrate lack of adequate understanding of HIV/AIDS. It seems to me that in order to control the epidemic, people should have more understanding of how the AIDS virus is passed on from one person to another and how it causes the disease AIDS.

Lack of understanding is one thing, but challenging the prevailing scientific basis of the disease is entirely another case. So-called AIDS dissidents have questioned the role of HIV in AIDS. In other words, they claim that HIV has nothing to do with AIDS; that is, the virus does not cause AIDS. It is truly mind-boggling to me that 20 years into the epidemic and more than 15 years after HIV was isolated, people would even question the relationship between the virus and AIDS. But these dissidents have been spreading their message, and unfortunately, some young people listening to those messages are not taking the necessary precautions they should to avoid getting the virus. Even worse is the fact that some policy makers are following that crusade and in the process putting their people's lives into jeopardy.

The biology of HIV disease is rather simple, following the classic germ theory. The germ theory involves parasite and host relationship. When a germ enters the body of another living organism, the germ (parasite) lives at the expense of the organism (host). Sometimes, there is a symbiotic relationship between the parasite and the host. In most cases, especially when the parasite enters a human, the relationship becomes an antagonistic one. The parasite often uses tissues and cells in the human for its survival. When cells and tissues are destroyed, the person may become ill. Often the host tries to fight the parasite; that is, there is a war between the parasite and host, and if the parasite wins, the host becomes ill. And depending upon other parameters and circumstances, the host may die. HIV is a particularly powerful parasite that always wins the war against its host, the human being.

When AIDS was first detected in homosexuals, it was thought that there was something unique about homosexual activity that caused the immune system breakdown. A similar assumption was made when AIDS started showing up in intravenous drug users. Finally, when AIDS was found at about equal rates in males and females in some African countries, the speculation was that a unique heterosexual activity by Africans promoted HIV transmission. The implication of all this is that just being homosexual, drug user, or African was a risk for AIDS.

I have always discounted the idea of risk groups vis-à-vis AIDS. The transmission of HIV is a biological phenomenon, and it is not based on group selection. Indeed, in my speeches, I make a blanket statement that getting AIDS has "nothing" to do sex or drug use. Then I explain further that AIDS is caused by a virus called HIV. The virus only needs to get into human tissue to cause cell destruction, leading to the disease AIDS.

The virus needs a pathway or route to enter the body tissues where it causes its cell destruction. *It uses any possible means* to get to that route. I maintain that the *route* of HIV transmission is blood; and the *means* of transmission (means of getting to blood) could be sexual, illicit drug injections, therapeutic drug injections, cuts on mucous membranes, cuts on the skin, blood transfusion, etc. In other words, one does not need to have sex or inject drugs to get AIDS; and one definitely does not have to have homosexual sex to get AIDS. The "H" in HIV does not stand for "homosexual"; it stands for "human". Therefore, if you are human, you can be infected by the Human Immunodeficiency Virus...under the right circumstances. On the other hand, it is not easy to acquire HIV, and people should not worry about so-called casual transmission.

The official policy regarding HIV transmission, as espoused by the U.S. Public Health Service and the World Health Organization, recognizes four means of HIV transmission: (1) sexual (both homosexual and heterosexual) activity, (2) intravenous (illicit) drug use, (3) transfusion of blood and blood products, and (4) from mother to child through the birth process and breast feeding. These four means of transmission have been emphasized from the beginning of the epidemic. So, when statistics are collected on AIDS cases, the figures are often listed by risk groups or exposure categories, using these four means of transmission. Though this process has value in tracking the epidemic, it confuses the issue when viewed outside scholarly circles. People in a statistically low risk group might think of themselves as being invulnerable to the disease and may not take serious action to avoid exposure to the virus.

Mechanism of HIV Transmission

The passing of an organism from an infected person to another person is referred to as *transmission*. Based upon basic microbiology and infectious disease principles, three factors must be satisfied for a successful transmission to occur: (1) there has to be a portal of exist, (2) there has to be a medium of survival, and (3) there has to be a portal of entry. Different organisms leave the body through different orifices and enter the next victim's body by another body organ.

Suppose a person with a cold sneezes with other people around. Hundreds of viruses are released from the person's nose (portal of exit); the viruses stay alive in the air for a few seconds (medium of survival); then a person close by breathes in the virus-saturated air through the nose and mouth (portal of entry). After achieving entry into the susceptible person's body, the viruses find their way into various body tissues where they establish themselves for procreation. At this stage, an infection has taken place. In the process of multiplying themselves, the viruses cause all kinds of damage to the tissues where they live, and this person develops the same cold symptoms as the original cold sufferer.

In the illustration above, when the cold sufferer sneezed and released so many viruses in the air, several people in the immediate vicinity would have been exposed to the same virus-saturated air. But not all of them would develop the same cold symptoms. This has to do with the fact that those who won the parasite-versus-host war would not become ill, and those who lost would. The ammunition used in this war by human beings is the immune system.

Viruses are paradoxical organisms. On one hand, they are fragile and delicate organisms that are nothing more than a package of genes inside a protein shell. They cannot live or reproduce on their own, and they use cells of other living organisms for survival and to reproduce themselves. In other words, they have no life and are obligate parasites. On the other hand, they can cause tremendous havoc, including death, to the organisms upon which their very survival depends. Different viruses use different types of cells of other living organisms for their living. Whether the relationship between a virus and its host is symbiotic or antagonistic depends upon the type of virus. And the relationship between HIV and human beings is an antagonistic one.

Viruses require precise sets of conditions to live. Therefore, some viruses thrive in cold climates, others in warm climates; some live in animal tissue, others prefer plant tissue; some can survive on surfaces of living organisms, others require entry into the body. In this regard, HIV is a special virus that requires entry into the body. All research evidence has demonstrated that HIV has to be transferred directly from an infected source to specialized cells in the human body for infection to occur. It goes to these cells by blood. Therefore, the often-repeated chorus that HIV is not transmitted through breathing, handshake, toilet seats, eating utensils, mosquitoes and other insects, is based on scientific evidence. Blood is the route of transmission of HIV, and it does not require sexual intercourse. How does blood relate to the four official means of transmission?

Transmission through sexual activity.

During heterosexual intercourse, HIV may be transmitted from the male to the female by semen or from the female to the male by vaginal fluid. In homosexual intercourse, the virus could be transmitted to the receptive partner by semen or the insertive partner by rectal fluid and blood. Whether exposure to the virus leads to transmission depends upon contact with blood by the virus, and it has nothing to do with the type of sexual act. The difference between the rate of infection through homosexual act and that of heterosexual has to do with the relative ease with which blood contact occurs.

The vagina is lined by a mucous membrane called *stratified squamous epithelium*. In the presence of normal lubrication, this epithelium is quite resistant to lacerations. In addition, the vaginal fluid is quite acidic, and HIV does not survive long in acidic environments. On the other hand, the rectal mucosa is lined be a membrane called *columnar epithelium*. This membrane is quite friable and breaks more easily. In addition, blood vessels are nearer to the surface of the anus, so membrane breakage leads to easy contact with blood. Furthermore, the anal opening is quite tight, and the insertion of an erect penis necessarily involves some degree of force, making lacerations much easier to occur. Therefore, though the portal of exist is similar in both acts, both medium of survival and portal of entry are more efficient in anal intercourse than in vaginal intercourse. And it has nothing to do with homosexuality. A woman receiving anal sex has as high a chance of HIV transmission as a man receiving anal sex.

The same principle is the reason for easier transmission from a man to a woman in heterosexual act. Studies have shown that in strictly heterosexual relationships, it is about 20 times easier for the man to transmit HIV to the woman than the reverse (Padien, et al, 1991). The act of sexual intercourse, with piston and socket kind of action, makes the vaginal mucosa break more easily. Though the vaginal mucosa is quite resilient, small breaks can and do occur during intercourse through which the virus can pass. Also, the vagina has a large surface area, and small breaks over a large area make for easy access to blood. In this regard, studies have shown that the reasons for the high male-to-female transmission rate include anal intercourse, bleeding during vaginal intercourse, and sex during the woman's menstrual period (Padien, et al; European Cooperative Study, 1992).

Another example of this phenomenon is the fact that there is a higher rate of HIV/AIDS among men who are not circumcised than those who are. Studies have shown that in countries where most of the men are circumcised, there is a relatively low prevalence of HIV/AIDS, and there is a much higher rate in the countries where most men are not circumcised (UNAIDS, 2001). The reason is that the foreskin provides a wider surface area for viruses to enter the body. Also, the uncircumcised penis is more likely to suffer small lacerations during intercourse; and the uncircumcised penis is more prone to genital ulcers and other sexually transmitted infections (STIs).

The discussion in the last couple of paragraphs indicates that HIV transmission through sexual intercourse depends upon how easily blood contact with the virus is achieved. It means that from male to female (and vice versa) or homosexual versus heterosexual should be similar if there is similar chance of blood contact. This is why people with STIs have high rates of HIV infection. Genital ulcers such as *chancre* (syphilis), *chancroid*, and genital herpes permit easy access to blood. Other STIs like *gonorrhoea*, *chlamydia*, and *trichomonas* produce inflammation that compromises the integrity of the vaginal, penal, and anal linings and creates access to blood. Thus the presence of STIs increases the chance of HIV transmission, whether it is in a male or female, heterosexual or homosexual. The very high rates of STIs in some African countries and other developing countries contribute to the high rates of HIV infection among heterosexuals in those countries.

The implication of the above discussion is that having sex with someone infected with HIV, male or female, will not necessarily result in transmission if there is no access of the virus to blood. But that is a very big if. Sustaining a mucosal break during sex is not difficult, particularly if sexual activity is frequent or involves several partners. Also, one can have genital ulcers or other STIs without knowing it. It necessarily follows that the more genital ulcers or other STIs there are, the more likely HIV transmission is. This leads to another principle of infectious disease: *dose and effect*.

This principle states that the higher the dose (of infective agent), the easier the transmission. High dose could result from a single exposure to a large number of viruses or frequent exposure to moderate number of viruses. As regards HIV, studies have shown that there are very high levels of the virus in the infected person during the early part of infection and the late stages of AIDS. Thus, transmission is more common at the early stages and when the infected person has AIDS. It is particularly dangerous at the early stages because the infected person may not know he or she is infected in order to abstain or use protection. Another principle of infectious disease, *mass action*, states that in the presence of a large number of viruses, transmission can occur even if there are only small mucosal breaks. Exposure to repeated penal pounding (causing mucosal breaks) and many different people (exposure to STIs) is one reason for the high rates of HIV infection among commercial sex workers or prostitutes. Of course, exposure to so many different people increases the chance of exposure to HIV.

Transmission through blood and blood products.

Based on the proposal above, blood transfusion should be, and it is, the easiest way for HIV transmission. Blood and blood products serve as both the portal of exist and medium of survival; and the portal of entry, the recipient's blood, is the most direct. Also important is dose effect. The transfusion of a pint of HIV infected blood introduces a large number of viruses at one time; and considering the fact that most transfusion recipients receive several pints of blood, this means is very efficient indeed. Therefore, there is about 90% to 100% chance that the transfusion of HIV infected blood or blood product would lead to HIV infection. This is why the rate of HIV infection among hemophiliacs used to be so high.

Hemophilia is a genetic disease in which the sufferer lacks certain clotting factors and is thus subjected to frequent bleeding. The patients survive by the transfusion of clotting factors that are pooled from the blood of hundreds of donors. In the earlier part of the AIDS epidemic, most of the clotting factors was contaminated by HIV, and 70% to 80% of hemophiliacs in the U.S. became infected with HIV. In more recent years, the infection rate is nearly zero because the factors are heat-treated before being transfused. Also since the development of blood tests to screen donated blood, transfusion-associated HIV transmission has virtually been eliminated in the U.S. and other developed countries. It is still a problem in some developing countries because of inadequate screening of donated blood.

Transmission through IV drug use.

Transmission of HIV through intravenous drug use is quite efficient because of blood, not the drug use itself. That is, it has to do with the sharing of needles, indeed the sharing of blood. Therefore, if one injects drugs and does not share equipment, there is no chance of contracting HIV. I have visited drug shooting galleries, and it is clear from what I observed that it is the sharing of blood that leads to HIV transmission.

When the drug users meet at those galleries, they undergo a ritual of mixing the drug with water and cooking it to dissolve the drug. Then the mixture is drawn into a syringe for injection. The first person inserts the needle in his or her vein, draws blood into the syringe, and then pushes the mixture of the blood and drug back into the vein. The syringe is passed on to the next person who does the same thing and passes it on to the next person, and so on. When the first person withdrew blood from his vein into the syringe and pushed it back into the vein, some droplets of blood remained in the syringe and on the tip of the needle. When the next person drew his blood into the syringe, it got mixed with the previous person's blood before being injected.

What happens here is the sharing of blood. Obviously, if the preceding blood is infected with HIV, it is transmitted to the succeeding users of the same syringe. As in the case of transfusions, blood is both the portal of exit and medium of survival, with a direct portal of entry. There may not be enough viruses injected at a time because of the small amount of blood involved, but the frequency with which drug users share needles makes for a very efficient means of transmission.

It should be emphasized that the drug use per se has nothing to do with HIV transmission if needle sharing is not involved. Studies in Britain, Switzerland, the Netherlands, Sweden and the United States have shown that when drug users are given unused syringes, the rate of HIV infection goes down among the drug users. Other studies in the United States have shown that even cleaning the syringes and needles with bleach between uses cuts down transmission. The reason, of course, is that no blood is shared when a clean syringe/needle is used be it brand new or a thoroughly washed used one.

Transmission from mother to child.

Most infants and small children with AIDS acquire HIV infection from their mothers during pregnancy or delivery. A woman with HIV infection or AIDS may transmit the virus to her foetus by means of maternal blood circulation during pregnancy or by blood inoculation during delivery. Transmission from mother to infant is, of course, very efficient since the mother shares blood circulation with the foetus. However, infected mothers do not always transmit the virus to the foetus. Earlier studies in the United States and Africa showed transmission rates of 30% to 50%. More recent studies found only 15% to 30% transmission rates.

When an infant tests positive for HIV antibodies at birth, it may not necessarily be from HIV infection. The mother could simply have passed on the antibodies to the foetus without passing on viruses. Maternal antibodies usually disappear from the infant's circulation after about age six months. Therefore, an infant with detectable antibody levels at birth should be monitored past six months; the blood test should turn negative after six months if no viruses were transmitted from the mother. However, it is recommended that the child be tested every three months until age 15 months, and if results are still negative, then the initial positive test is presumed to have come from maternal antibodies. In any case, the child with the virus often develops symptoms of HIV infection quite early after birth, often before 15 months of age. Researchers are not sure why 100% of infected mothers do not pass on the virus to their infants. It may be related to the degree of the mother's illness; transmission rates are high when the mother has high p24 antigen (viral particles) levels, low T4 cell levels in her blood, and placental membrane inflammation (St. Louis, et al, 1993).

The mother with HIV infection can also pass the virus on to her infant through breast-feeding. Again, just as through the birth process, the chance of passing it through breast-feeding is not 100%; the chance is 10% to 20%. In this regard, the WHO recommends that HIV-infected mothers in some developing countries may breast feed their infants since the chance of dying from diarrhoeal diseases as a result of not breast feeding may be higher than that of acquiring HIV infection through breast milk.

I stated at the beginning of this chapter that I have discounted the idea of risks and exposure categorization regarding HIV transmission. This is because such a system does not tell the full story. There are other means than the four official ones of HIV transmission. Furthermore, when "risk groups" is used to label means of transmission, it confuses matters. It tends to reinforce the notion that only certain types of people get AIDS. This, of course, can produce stigmatisation of certain people, in addition to creating a false sense of invulnerability on the part of those who do not fall into the risk groups.

So, it is worth repeating that HIV transmission can occur by any means as long as there is access to blood by the virus. Transmission has occurred through cuts on mucous membranes, cuts on the skin, and even cracks on the skin. These have occurred mostly among health care workers who were splashed with infected blood accidentally. Also, transmission has occurred with accidental needle-stick of health care workers.

The frequency of transmission through these latter means is much lower than those discussed earlier because of dose effect. There is usually very little blood involved with accidental needle-sticks. There could be a significant time lapse between when the needle leaves the infected person and when the accidental stick occurs; the virus may not survive that long. Also, the needle-stick may not be deep enough for blood exposure. So, most needle-stick injuries and blood splashes do not result in HIV transmission. Even when workers have stuck themselves with needles known to be contaminated with HIV infected blood, the rate of transmission is still low. Studies from the U.S. National Institutes of Health have shown the rate of HIV transmission by a single needle-stick injury to be 0.46%.

Can casual transmission of HIV occur? The answer depends upon how one defines "casual". If casual transmission refers to means other than the four official ones, then the answer is absolutely yes...as discussed in the last paragraphs. If casual transmission means through handshakes, food or drink, toilet seats, sharing cooking and eating utensils, mosquitoes and other insect bites, then the answer is no. However, it is better to avoid such labels as "casual" and "intimate" in discussing transmission. There is nothing intimate about receiving HIV infected blood transfusion. On the other hand, "casual" transmission can occur as is possible from splashes or needle-stick with infected blood.

What about transmission through kissing and spitting? There is no question that HIV has been isolated from saliva, as it has been from other body fluids like breast milk, tears, urine and cerebrospinal fluid. However, the concentration of HIV in these body fluids is too low for effective transmission (dose effect). Except for that of breast-feeding as discussed above, there have been no reported cases of HIV transmission through the other body fluids.

A study reported by researchers at the U.S. National Institute of Dental Research demonstrated that not only is saliva not a major source of HIV infection, it might actually be protective. They incubated HIV in saliva with lymphocytes, and the lymphocytes were completely protected from infection. Even when they diluted the saliva at 1:20, it was still 50% protective. The researchers concluded that there might be "a natural, non toxic product" in saliva that may have "potential therapeutic benefits" (Fettrer, 1990).

Pathogenesis of AIDS

The mechanism of disease progression, how exposure to a causative agent leads to development of disease, is referred to as *pathogenesis*. Acquired Immunodeficiency Syndrome (AIDS) results from the inability or impaired ability of the body's immune system to do its job of protecting against various diseases. In other words, the immune system is deficient hence the name *immunodeficiency*. A syndrome is a collection of symptoms or illnesses with a common cause. Thus, AIDS is not really a disease but a number of different diseases all resulting from one cause (deficient immune system). Though AIDS is a new condition, there is nothing new about immune deficiency in medical science.

Some people are born with various degrees of immune system impairment; that is, parts of the system are functional and other parts are impaired. Such people are unable to fight off certain specific infections but are able to survive quite well. Childhood diseases such as *Di George Syndrome, Bruton's Disease*, and *Chedak-Higashi Syndrome* all involve immune system impairment. However, total lack of immune system function is incompatible with life. A condition called *Combined Immune System Disease* (CIDS) results from total lack of immune system function, and children with this condition often die early in childhood from simple infections that are otherwise not dangerous.

The significant thing about immune deficiency is that it does not kill its victims directly but leaves them vulnerable to both simple and serious infections. Therefore, a child with CIDS could live a full lifespan if it were protected from exposure to infectious agents.

A child called David was a CIDS patient in Houston, Texas in the United States in 1970s. He was kept in a sterile plastic bubble soon after birth, so he had no physical contact to people or contaminated objects. He lived in the bubble for 12 years, at which time he received a bone marrow transplant. The transplant was unsuccessful, and he died after being taken out of the bubble. AIDS is similar to CIDS, except in the case of AIDS, the person is born with an intact immune system. He or she acquires something (hence the name *acquired*) that destroys the immune system to the point of being vulnerable to simple and serious infections. Again, acquiring immune deficiency is nothing new.

Acquired immune deficiency can be caused by certain chemotherapeutic medications, corticosteroid, certain types of cancer, and kidney disease with the consequent risk for infections. In most of these cases the immune deficiency is not complete, and such infections are often managed with aggressive antibiotic treatment. And the immune deficiency is usually resolved when the inciting medication or illness is eliminated. The unique thing about AIDS is that the immune deficiency is caused by a virus (HIV), and the immune system destruction is to the extent that antibiotics are often not able to cure the resulting infections. How does HIV cause the immune deficiency? Before answering that question, a discussion of the human immune system is in order.

As human beings, we are surrounded by all kinds of dangerous organisms or germs. These organisms do not kill us because of a powerful protective mechanism called the immune system. Indeed, we are protected by two major barriers; the skin and mucous membranes provide the first line of defence, and the immune system comes into play when the organism enters the body.

Most organisms cannot penetrate the intact skin, and all the other orifices of the body are lined by mucous membranes that cannot be penetrated by most organisms. When the integrity of the skin or mucous membrane is compromised, certain organisms may enter the body. Once the organisms enter the body, the various ammunitions of the immune system are called upon to fight the invaders, much as the military of a country is called upon to fight foreign invaders. The immune system responds in a similar way when any foreign object enters the body such as pollen, dust, and some types of food in people who have allergic sensitivity.

Organisms usually travel through the lymphatic channels to the bloodstream and then to various tissues in the body. There is the phenomenon of *tissue trophism*; that is, different organisms prefer different body tissue. Some organisms stay outside cells, others invade and stay inside cells. The organisms may be destroyed in the lymphatic channel, but if they reach the bloodstream, they are attacked by circulating cells called *phagocytes*. If they are able to reach tissue, tissue phagocytes called *macrophages* attack them. At this stage, more ammunition in the immune system is called upon.

Special white blood cells called *lymphocytes* come to the aid of the macrophages in the destruction of the organisms. Whether the body is able to conquer the organisms depends upon the number (dose effect) and the virulence (the strength) of the organism versus the number and quality of the human cells doing the fighting. If the body "loses the war", the organisms set up housekeeping and cause damage to tissue or cells. The person may then develop symptoms characteristic of the disease caused by that particular organism. If the body wins the war, the person may not know he or she has been attacked.

There are two types of lymphocytes: *B-lymphocytes* and *T-lymphocytes* (or B cells and T cells). The lymphocytes form the backbone of the immune system; and in general the B cells fight organisms outside cells, while the T cells attack organisms that invade cells. The B cells produce antibodies that destroy bacteria, and the T cells destroy viruses, parasites, and fungi. But the production of antibodies by the B cells requires the assistance of T cells.

There are three main types of T cells: natural killer cells, T-helper cells (T4), and T-suppressor cells (T8). Natural killer cells are scavenger cells that roam and destroy foreign objects. The T-suppressor cells protect normal human cells from being attacked by the body's own immune cells. The T-helper cells are the most important of all the immune cells. They are the cells required by the B cells for antibody production. They also assist the phagocytic cells, direct destruction of organisms, and direct antibody production by the T cell system—hence its name *helper*. In effect, the whole immune system is dependent upon the T-helper cells. And the body uses the T cell system to fight all viral infections with considerable degree of success, but it is a different story regarding HIV.

The human immunodeficiency virus (HIV), like all other viruses, is an *obligate intracellular organism;* that is, it must enter cells to survive. It belongs to a group of viruses called *retroviruses*. It is an RNA (ribonucleic acid) virus. All organisms require DNA (deoxyribonucleic acid) to reproduce themselves, so retroviruses should not be able to reproduce. However, HIV has a special enzyme called *reverse transcriptase* with which it works backwards (reverse to the usual process) to reproduce itself. But it requires human cells to do that. Once inside the human cell, it uses reverse transcriptase to convert its RNA into a DNA particle called *provirus*. The provirus is integrated into the DNA of the infected person's (host) cell. The host cell is no more a human cell, and it produces a new RNA (HIV) virus. In other words, the retrovirus impregnates the host cell to give birth to another retrovirus. In the process, the host cell dies. Sometimes the virus lies dormant in the host cell but the host cell is forever infected.

The paradox of HIV infection, which makes it so dangerous, is that of all the numerous types of cells in the human body, HIV selectively uses T4 (T-helper cell), the most important of the immune cells, to reproduce itself. This is because like all viruses, it requires a specific site on the host cell for attachment, and its preferred site is called CD4. The CD4 molecule is found most abundantly on T4 cells; it is also found in smaller quantities on macrophages, brain cells, and gut cells called *chromafin cells*.

Once HIV infects an individual, its progressive destruction of T4 cells is relentless. Antibodies are made against HIV but they are not effective in killing the viruses because of the destruction of T4 (helper) cells. So, the virus keeps reproducing itself and killing CD4 cells until the host does not have enough cells to protect itself, at which time illnesses characteristic of AIDS may develop. The average adult human has about 1000 CD4 cells per decilitre of blood serum, with a range of about 500 to 1700. When the CD4 cell count drops to below 200, the host is unable to fight infections by common and unusual organisms and develops AIDS symptoms. Under some circumstances such as the presence of other diseases, AIDS symptoms may occur at CD4 above 200 but very rarely above 500.

The progression from HIV infection to AIDS depends upon how fast CD4 cells are destroyed based on individual characteristics. The rate of destruction depends upon the number of viruses versus the number and quality of CD4 cells in the body. Also, lymphocytes that have been chronically stimulated, because of infection by other organisms, are infected and destroyed more easily by HIV (Quinn, et al, 1987). Indeed, the status of the whole immune system depends upon the general health of the individual, nutritional status, environmental stress, and existence of other diseases. Therefore, a person with HIV infection is likely to develop AIDS in a relatively short time if:

(1)   he or she has poor general health
(2)   he or she has poor nutritional status
(3)   he or she is under a lot of environmental stress
(4)   he or she has coexisting illnesses, particularly
        certain infectious diseases that tend to stimulate
        the immune system.

Because of the dose effect versus host status, different people develop AIDS at different times after HIV infection. Studies have shown that about 50% of people with HIV infection would develop AIDS within seven to ten years, and 100% would get it in 19 years. However, it is not easy to tell who will get it in less than

10 years and who will go for 19 years without AIDS. It all depends upon how healthy the person is before HIV infection, the dose of infection, and how the person cares for himself or herself once infection has taken place.

I have discussed this phenomenon in my oral presentations with what I call the "dam theory". A dam is erected to hold water at bay. Rain could cause flooding on the other side of the dam based on the height of the dam and intensity of the rain:

(1)   If it rains in very large amounts and the dam is relatively short, there will be flooding.

(2)   If it rains in very large amounts and the dam is relatively tall, there could be flooding.

(3)   If it rains in moderate amounts and the dam is relatively short, there will be flooding.

(4)   If it rains in moderate amounts and the dam is relatively tall, there will be no flooding.

The dam theory may help explain why some people take a long time to develop AIDS after HIV infection and others get AIDS rather quickly. People with relatively tall dams (strong immune system) and moderate rain (moderate number of viruses) may take a long time to develop AIDS. On the other hand those with relatively short dams (weak immune system) but large amount of rain (large number of viruses) can get AIDS quite quickly. The dam theory applies irrespective of group or individual characteristics. Whether through homosexual or heterosexual encounter, whether through blood transfusion or IV drug use, one is likely to get AIDS quickly if "the amount of rain is large enough to cause flooding."

Clinical Manifestations of AIDS

Once a person is infected with HIV, there is a progression from initial infection to full-blown AIDS. The initial HIV infection may or may not produce flu-like symptoms—headache, body aches, fatigue, fever, and so on. These same symptoms could be present with other viral illnesses, so a doctor may not think about HIV infection, especially if the patient is not from a so-called risk group. The flu-like illness may last a few days with complete recovery. As more lymphocytes are destroyed, the patient may develop symptoms characteristic of ARC (AIDS - related complex) and finally AIDS. Some people may not have the initial flu-like symptoms or ARC; they are diagnosed with full-blown AIDS at the first presentation for medical care. Others may remain in asymptomatic state or go from ARC to persistent generalized lymphadenopathy (see Figure 3). A person with at least two of the following is considered to have ARC:

(1)   unexplained lymphadenopathy (swollen lymph nodes in various parts of the body).

(2)   fever of unknown origin for at least three weeks

(3)   unexplained diarrhoea resulting in weight loss of at least 10 kilograms

(4)   unexplained fatigue for at least three weeks.

The development of AIDS occurs when the immune destruction is well advanced. In this regard, the illnesses that define AIDS— illnesses that are normally benign in people with intact immune system—start appearing when the CD4 count falls below 200. The following clinical conditions formed the qualifying definition of AIDS during the early part of the epidemic:

(1)   unusual cancers
      a. Kaposi's sarcoma
      b. some types of lymphomas
(2)   constitutional symptoms
      a. fever, decreased (or lack of) appetite, fatigue, weight loss
      b. opportunistic infections
(3)   AIDS dementia or HIV encephalopathy.

The above definition of AIDS was a bit restrictive. It was revised in 1987 to include more patients who might otherwise not fit the definition. In August 1987, the CDC issued the revised definition of AIDS that stated that a person with a positive HIV antibody test and at least one of 23 conditions had AIDS (see Table 3). In October 1992, the CDC added the following to the 23 conditions: (1) pulmonary tuberculosis, (2) recurrent pneumonia, (3) invasive cervical cancer, and (4) CD4 level less than 200. Regarding (4), it means that a person with CD4 cell level below 200 has AIDS whether or not he or she has any of the 26 AIDS-defining illnesses.

Table 3. REVISED DEFINITION OF AIDS (CDC, 1987)

Candidiasis—bronchial, trachea, lungs
Candidiasis—oesophageal
Coccidioiodomycosis—disseminated or extra pulmonary
Cryptococcosis—extra pulmonary
Cryptosporidiosis—chronic intestinal
Cytomegalovirus—retinitis with vision loss
Cytomegalovirus—other than liver, spleen, nodes
Herpes simples—chronic ulcers
Histoplasmosis—disseminated or extra pulmonary
HIV encephalopathy (AIDS dementia)
Isosporiasis—chronic intestinal Kaposi's sarcoma
Lymphoma—Burkitt's or equivalent
Lymphoma—primary in brain
Lymphoma—immunoblastic or equivalent
Mycobacterium tuberculosis—disseminated or extra
pulmonary
Mycobacterium avium—disseminated or extra pulmonary
Mycobacterium—other, disseminated or extra pulmonary
Pneumocystis carinii pneumonia (PCP)
Progressive multifocal leukoencephalopathy
Salmonella septicaemia, recurrent Toxoplasmosis of the
brain
Wasting syndrome—weight loss of more than 10% baseline
Weight loss and diarrhoea or fatigue.

SOURCE: U.S. Centers for Disease Control (1987).

The new 1992 definition was expected to increase the number of reported AIDS cases by at least 10% by the addition of the new diseases. With this in mind some AIDS experts have argued that the breakdown of the disease into HIV infection, ARC, and AIDS is confusing. The terms ARC and AIDS should be dropped and *HIV disease* be adopted since progression from infection to full-blown AIDS is a continuum. However, for logistic purposes and

```
                              Continuing              Persistent
                            Asymptomatic             Generalized
                                  State          Lymphadenopathy
                                    ↗                    ↗
HIV        →  Development  →  Asymptomatic  →  ARC
Infection     of Antibodies   Carrier State          ↘
                                                      AIDS
```

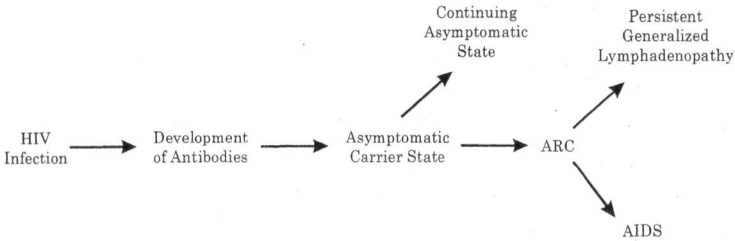

for familiarity sake, AIDS will always be used to define the terminal stages of the disease. But ARC has all but been eliminated from the lexicon of the HIV/AIDS epidemic.

Laboratory check of CD4 count is central to the CDC definition in diagnosing AIDS and making decisions about when to start treatment. Obviously, this had limitations in that it is not possible to do CD4 counts in many developing countries because of lack of the technology and trained personnel to do the test, and the cost involved. Therefore, the World Health Organization (WHO) came up with a simplified staging system that is clinically based.

The WHO has put the progression of HIV disease into four stages. Stage 1 (Asymptomatic stage) signifies a person with HIV infection and virtually no symptom; in Stage 2 (Early disease stage) the patient has very few symptoms; stage 3 (intermediate disease stage) is when the patient displays many diseases related to AIDS; and in Stage 4 (severe disease stage) the patient is often very sick with severe diseases. The clinical staging helps clinicians in resource-poor areas monitor the patient's progress in order to make treatment decisions. In stages 1 and 2, the patients may be seen less often than in stages 3 and 4 during which very close monitoring is essential. Also, most clinicians would decide to place patients on ARV only when they have reached Stage 3 or Stage 4.

This does not mean that those in earlier stages should never be placed on ARV but rather in light of the side effects and cost, those at the latter stages should have priority. The following is an outline of the WHO staging system:

WHO Stage 1— **Asymptomatic stage:**
Asymptomatic HIV infection
Persistent generalized lymphadenopathy (PGL)

WHO Stage 2— **Early stage:**
Herpes zoster within the last year
Minor mucocutaneous manifestation
Recurrent upper respiratory tract infections
Weight loss less than or equal to 10%

WHO Stage 3— **Intermediate (moderate disease) stage:**
Severe bacterial infections (pneumonia, pyomyositis)
Oral candidiasis (thrush)
Unexplained chronic diarrhoea (more than one month)
Unexplained prolonged fever (more than one month)
Oral hairy leukoplasia
Pulmonary tuberculosis (within the previous year
Weight loss more than 10% body weight

WHO Stage 4—	Late (severe disease) stage:
	Candidiasis (oesophageal, bronchi, trachea, lung)
	Cryptococcosis, extra pulmonary
	Cryptosporidiosis with diarrhoea more than one month
	Cytomegalovirus disease (other than spleen, lympnodes)
	Herpes simplex (mucocuteneaous more than one month or visceral, any duration)
	HIV encephalopathy
	HIV wasting syndrome
	Kaposi's sarcoma
	Lymphoma
	Atypical Mycobacteria,
	disseminated Mycosis, disseminated endemic (e.g. histoplasmosis, coccidiodomycosis)
	Tuberculosis, extra-pulmonary;
	pneumocystis carinii
	pneumonia (PCP)
	Progressive mutifocal leukoencephalopathy (PML)
	Salmonella septicaemia, non-typhoid
	Toxoplasmosis, CNS

Why is AIDS so fatal? Why do some people survive with AIDS longer than others? During the 1980s the average length of time from AIDS diagnosis to death was about 36 months; it is much longer now largely because of more effective therapies. But most people with AIDS will die within seven to ten years. Obviously, how long one has AIDS before diagnosis plays a role in how long one survives with the disease. However, in general, the rapid downward course of AIDS has to do the immune system; that is, the inability to fight off common and unusual organisms.

There are four main microbial groups—bacteria, viruses, fungi, and parasites. The immune system protects us from these organisms, particularly the viruses, fungi, and parasites. With an intact immune system, our bodies are able to fight off infections by organisms from those three groups such that we often do not know that we have been infected. Bacterial infections, on the other hand, often result in illness that is usually treated successfully with anti-microbial medications (antibiotics). Regardless of the type of organism, successful treatment with anti-microbial drugs depends upon the immune system.

The microorganisms are living organisms as we humans are. Therefore, the anti-microbial drugs could kill us if given in high enough concentrations. We are usually given low doses of the medicine but enough to kill the microorganisms without killing us. The medicines kill most of the organisms, and then the body's immune system takes over and completes the destruction of the organisms for a cure. In other words, a successful cure of microbial infections by anti-microbial drugs requires the help of the immune system.

People with AIDS, of course, have no effective immune system. Thus, they require higher doses of anti-microbial drugs, often given intravenously. They eventually die from the infections because their bodies do not have the immune system to complete the cure, so they only get better instead of getting cured. They are often in and out of hospitals until they die. How quickly they die has to do with the status of the immune system before HIV infection and other factors discussed earlier in this chapter. So it is very difficult to treat opportunistic infections. It is even more difficult to treat HIV infection itself because of the tricky nature of getting medicine into human cells to kill HIV without killing the human cells.

Conclusion

I have tried in this chapter to shed more light on the biology of HIV infection and AIDS. HIV is a unique virus that is not transmitted easily, which is very fragile but whose infection leads to a devastating disease. It requires living cells to survive and reproduce itself. It is not transmitted through the air, from inanimate objects, by mosquitoes or other insects. Once exposure has occurred, transmission is through blood. Thus, any possible contact of the virus with blood by any means is a risk for HIV transmission. Therefore, we should refrain from labelling people as risk groups. Every human being is at risk for HIV infection...under the right circumstances.

With this in mind, we should stop worrying about so-called casual transmission. A former U.S. Surgeon General, C. Everett Koop, said some people could not get HIV even if they tried. I disagree slightly with that assertion; I say people almost have to try to get HIV. In other words, people have to indulge in specific activities and behaviours in order to contract HIV infection. Thus, we should all try to avoid those activities that put us at risk, and then we would not have to worry about getting AIDS. Health care professionals have adopted the concept of "universal precautions"; that is, viewing every sample of blood or body fluid as potentially infectious of HIV...and other blood borne organisms. We should all adopt that principle by viewing every human being as a potential carrier of HIV and take the necessary precautions in every situation where contact to or exchange of blood and other bodily fluids is possible.

We should understand how HIV invades human cells with particular affinity for T4 cells, the most important cell in the immune system. It enters T4 cells and commandeers them to reproduce itself by integrating itself into the human cell's DNA. In this regard it is difficult to get medicine to kill HIV without killing the cells. Besides, there are many strains of HIV; the virus undergoes frequent mutation, and it develops resistance to antiviral drugs. These factors make it difficult to develop effective drugs and vaccines for HIV.

We should bear in mind that all viruses invade cells in order to cause infection. Because of that no viral infection has ever been cured in history including the viruses that cause the common cold. A few drugs have been produced to treat, not cure, some viral infections, examples being *Acyclovir* for herpes, *Amantadine* for influenza A, *Riboviran* for influenza B, and AZT and other antiretroviral medications for HIV. All these drugs make the particular viral infection less severe than it might otherwise be; they do not cure the infections. If scientists have not been able find a cure for the common cold in hundreds of years, why are they chastised for not finding a cure for a complex virus like HIV in 20 years? We should not hold our breaths for a cure soon.

REFERENCES

1. Centers for Disease Control (1987). Revision of the surveillance case definition for acquired immunodeficiency syndrome. *MMWR*, 36, Sl-S15.

2. European Collaborative Study (1991). Children born to women with HIV-1 infection: natural history and risk of transmission. *Lancet*, 338, 253-260.

3. European Study Group on Heterosexual Transmission of HIV (1992). Comparison of female-to-male and male-to female transmission of HIV in 563 stable couples. *British Medical Journal*, 304, 809-813.

4. Fettrer, A.C. (1990, October 4). Saliva may inhibit HIV. *Medical Tribune,* p. 109.

5. Fischl, M.A., et al (1987). Evaluation of heterosexual partners, children, and household contacts of adults with AIDS. *Journal of American Medical Association*, 257, 640-644.

6. Francis, D.P., et al (1985). The natural history of infection with the lymphadenopathy-associated virus/human T-lymphotrophic virus type-III. *Annals of Internal Medicine*, 103, 719-722.

7. Friedland, G.H., et al (1986). Lack of transmission of HTLV-III\LAV infection to household contacts with AIDS-related complex with oral candidiasis. *New England Journal of Medicine*, 314, 344-349.

8. Fries, J.F., et al (1993). Effect of the new 1993 criteria for classification of AIDS. *Journal of American Medical Association*, 269, 2846-2847.

9. Ho, D.D., et al (1985). Infrequency of HTLV III virus from saliva in AIDS. *New England uJournal of Medicine*, 313, 1606.

10. Mann, J.M., et al (1986). Prevalence of HTLV-III\LAV in household contacts of patients with confirmed AIDS and controls in Kinshasa, Zaire. *Journal of American Medical Association*, 256, 721-724.

11. Matthew, T.J. & Bolognesi, D.P. (1988). AIDS vaccines. *Scientific American*, 259, 120-127.

12. Morse, S.S. & Brown, R.D. (1993). The enemy within. *Modern Maturity* 36, 50-54.

13. Oksenhendler, E., (1986). HIV infection with sero-conversion after a superficial needle-stick injury to the finger. *New England Journal of*

Medicine, 315, 582.

14. Padian, N.S., et al (1991). Female-to-male transmission of human immunodeficiency virus. *Journal of American Medical Association,* 1664-1667.

15. Piot, P. & Colebunders, R. (1987). Clinical manifestations and the natural history of HIV infection in adults. *Western Medical Journal,* 147, 709-712.

16. Quinn, T.C., et al (1987). Serologic and immunologic studies in patients with AIDS in North America and Africa: the potential role of infectious agents as co-factor in human immunodeficiency virus infection. *Journal of American Medical Association,* 257, 2089-2093.

17. Redfield, R.R. & Burke, D.S. (1988). HIV infection: the clinical picture. *Scientific American,* 259, 11

18. St. Loius, M.E., et al (1993). Risk for perinatal HIV-1 transmission according to maternal immunologic, virologic, and placental factors. *Journal of American Medical Association,* 269, 2853-2859.

19. Vergilio, J-A, et al (1993). The risk of exposure of third year surgical students to human immunodeficiency virus in the operating room. *Archives of Surgery,* 128, 36-39.

20. Weber, J.N. & Weiss, R. (1988). HIV infection; the cellular picture. *Scientific American,* 259, 101-109.

21. Winkelstein, W., et al (1987). Sexual practices and risk of infection by human immunodeficiency virus: the San Francisco Men's Study Group. *Journal of American Medical Association,* 257, 32I-325.

22. Yarchoan, R., et al (1988). AIDS therapies. *Scientific American,* 259, 110-119.

CHAPTER FOUR

MANAGEMENT OF HIV/AIDS

Everyone knows (or should know) that there is no cure for AIDS. Until antiviral medications were developed, most AIDS patients died within a few years of developing full-blown AIDS. They died from one or more of the numerous opportunistic diseases that characterize AIDS. Management of AIDS patients then involved treating opportunistic infections, which was really a temporary measure; they ultimately succumbed to the disease. How long one lived after AIDS diagnosis depended upon one's access to the medications to treat the opportunistic infection, along with other individual characteristics such nutritional and general health status.

With the introduction of antiviral medications, the management of HIV/AIDS became two-fold: (1) to treat those with HIV infection but not full-blown AIDS so as to delay the onset of AIDS symptoms for as long as possible; and (2) to treat AIDS patients so that they might live as long and as healthfully as possible. Here the treatment is with both antiviral medications and drugs to treat opportunistic infections. These were the goals of HIV/AIDS management for the first 15 years of the epidemic. Even with the antiviral medications, the patients ultimately died. Then the protease inhibitors were introduced in 1996, and people started talking about a cure for HIV/AIDS. But alas after a few years of experience with the protease inhibitors, it became clear that they are no cure. We were back to square one.

Like the treatment of opportunistic infections, that with antiviral medications involves "the haves and have-nots". These medications are very expensive. Therefore, whereas many patients in wealthy countries can avail themselves of these medications, they remain a dream for most patients in poorer countries. In wealthier nations, individuals with money are able to purchase the drugs or acquire insurance for the purchase, and those without the means are often get medicines that are subsidized by their governments. However, even in the rich countries, a segment of the population does not have access to the medications because of poverty. Nowhere is the adage "you cannot afford to be sick" more relevant than in the world of HIV/AIDS.

AIDS advocates, particularly those in developing countries, and governments in the poorer countries have decried the phenomenon. They have asked and even demanded that the drug companies reduce the prices for these drugs so all HIV/AIDS patients everywhere can afford them. For example, Dr. Peter Piot, executive director of UNAIDS, stated at a forum in November 2000 in Brazil that it was unacceptable that drugs should be beyond the reach of some people and some countries. He added: "We cannot tolerate a world where some regions have access to life-saving treatments and others are excluded, or societies where some classes of the population have comprehensive care but others have no chance of access." (AIDSLinks, 2000; p.7).

AIDS advocates have been appealing to drug companies for years to lower their prices, yet by the end of the year 2000, the drugs were largely out of reach to 95% of people with HIV/AIDS worldwide. But as the pressure on the drug companies continued, they seemed to be taking small steps to rectify the situation. For example, Glaxo-Wellcome, one of the leading manufacturers of HIV/AIDS medications made a deal with the government of Senegal in October 2000 to offer three of its medications (Retrovir, Epivir, and Combivir) at about US$2 a day. This formed part of a gesture made earlier by five drug companies to provide more affordable drugs to Africa (AIDSLink, 2000). Ironically, Senegal has one the lowest HIV/AIDS prevalence rates in Africa.

As the pressure on the drug companies mounted, they finally succumbed and announced in March 2001 that they would make the drugs available in the developing countries at about one-tenth the cost in the developed countries. These medicines cost about US$10,000 to US$15,000 a year; and when the costs of other medicines used for opportunistic diseases plus doctor visits and blood tests are added, the cost of managing patients approaches US$20,000 a year. So 10% of the cost in the developed world is still a lot more than most individuals and even governments in some of these countries could afford. Even the US$2 a day gesture to Senegal amounts to US$60 a month for three medications only. When one adds other costs to the care of an HIV/AIDS patient such as drugs to treat opportunistic infections, drug therapy still remains a dream for most HIV/AIDS in the world.

Management With Antiviral Medications

As discussed in the last chapter, 16 drugs were available to treat HIV/AIDS by the end of the year 2000. They fell into three classes—nucleoside reverse transcriptase inhibitors (NRTIs), non-nucleoside reverse transcriptase inhibitors NNRTIs), and protease inhibitors (PIs). They all work by preventing HIV from successfully reproducing itself. The NRTIs and NNRTIs work at the earlier stages of the virus's reproductive cycle, and the PIs work at the final stage when the new virus is leaving the human cell to invade other cells.

In light of their mechanism of action, combination therapy with medications from two or all three classes is more effective in getting rid of the virus. Also, the virus is less likely to develop drug resistant strains when combination therapy is employed. However, combination therapy is more problematic in terms of cost, number of pills to take at a time (pill burden), and side effects (Jacobson & Hicks, 2000). Other problems with antiviral medications involve multiple dosing, whether or not to take with food, and drug-drug interactions (see table 4.1). In addition, patients with full-blown AIDS may have to take other medications to prevent or treat opportunistic infections, and that increases the chance of side effects and drug-drug interactions. Thus a person with full-blown AIDS on antiviral medications and medications for opportunistic infections would have to contend with cost, pill burden, side effects, and lifestyle restrictions.

Table 4.1   Approved Antiretroviral Medications as of December, 2000

a) Nucleoside Reverse Transcriptase Inhibitors (NRTIs)

DRUG NAME	DOSING	FOOD RESTRICTIONS	SIDE EFFECTS
Zidovudine (Retrovir, AZT	200mg 3x/day or 300mg 2x/day (6 pills/day)	None	Leucopoenia, anaemia, fatigue, malaise, headache, hepatitis, myopathy, lactic acidosis
Didanosine (Videx, ddI)	200mg 2x/day (4 pills/day)	1 hour before meal	Headache, abdominal pain, lactic acidosis, pancreatitis
Stavudine (Zerit, d4T)	40mg 2x/day (2 pills/day	None	Peripheral neuropathy, nausea, vomiting, lactic acidosis
Lamivudine (Epivir, 3TC)	150mg 2x/day (2 pills/day)	None	Headache, insomnia, rash, lactic acidosis
Lamivudine/Zidovudine (Combivir)	1 pill 2x/day (2 pills/day)	None	Fever, rash, nausea, vomiting, lactic acidosis
Abacavir (Ziagin, ABC)	300mg 2x/day (2 pills/day	Avoid alcohol	Leucopoenia, anaemia, fatigue, headache

b) Non-nucleoside Reverse Transcriptase Inhibitors (NNRTIS):

DRUG NAME	DOSING	FOOD RESTRICTIONS	SIDE EFFECTS
Delavirdine (Rescriptor, DLV)	400mg 3x/day (6 pills/day)	Avoid antacids	Rash, Steven-Johnson syndrome, elevated liver enzymes
Efavirenz (Sustiva, EFV)	600mg at bedtime (3 pill/day)	Avoid high fat meals	Rash, Steven-Johnson syndrome, nightmares, hallucinations, mood disturbances
Nevirapine (Viramune, NVP)	200mg 1x/day for two weeks, then 200mg 2x/day (2 pills/day)	None	Rash, Steven-Johnson syndrome, elevated liver enzymes

c) Protease Inhibitors (PIs)

Nelfinavir (Viracept, NFV)	750mg 3x/day (9 pills/day	Take with food	Diarrhoea, hyperglycaemia, fat redistribution, abnormal lipids
Indanavir (Crixivan, IDV)	800mg 3x/day (6 pills/day)	1 hour before or 2 hours after meals	Kidney stones, nausea, headache, dizziness, hyperglycaemia, fat redistribution, abnormal lipids
Ritonavir (Norvir, RTV)	600mg 2x/day (6 pills/day)	Take with food	Nausea, vomiting, diarrhoea, peripheral neuropathy, fat redistribution, abnormal lipids
Sanquinavir (Fortovase, SQV)	1200mg 3x/day (18 pills/day)	Take with food	Nausea, vomiting, diarrhoea, headache, hyperglycaemia, fat redistribution, abnormal lipids
Sanquinavir (Invirase)	600mg 3x/day (9 pills/day)	None	Nausea, vomiting, diarrhoea, headache, hyperglycaemia, fat redistribution, abnormal lipids
Amprenavir (Agenerase, PAV)	1200mg 2x/day (16 pills/day)	Avoid high fat meals	Nausea, vomiting, diarrhoea, rash, hyperglycaemia, fat redistribution, abnormal lipids

SOURCE: Glaxo Wellcome

How is it decided when and in whom to start antiviral medications? As discussed in the last chapter, CD4 count and viral load are a marker of disease progression. In other words, low CD4 count and high viral load indicate bad clinical status, and high CD4 count and low viral load indicate good clinical status. The goal of medical treatment, therefore, is to increase the CD4 count as much as possible and decrease the viral load, preferably to below the level of laboratory detection.

Before 1996, people with advanced HIV disease usually died in two to three years from opportunistic infections. They were treated with one or two NRTIs or NNRTIs. These medications could not suppress the levels of HIV for long periods of time; and in addition to problems with drug resistance, they were not very effective in controlling the disease. With the introduction of the PIs in 1996, HIV/AIDS patients started feeling much better and living longer. Combination therapy with the protease inhibitors and reverse transcriptase inhibitors was found to be very effective in treating the disease. The combination was named *Highly Active Antiretroviral Therapy* (HAART).

The term HAART refers to a regimen of three or more antiretroviral medications that can suppress HIV to very low or undetectable levels for long periods of time. In addition to preventing disease progression, HAART was to prevent the emergence of resistance strains of the virus (Jacobson & Hicks, 2000). As stated in the last chapter, the use of PIs (in HAART) led to the decline of deaths from HIV/AIDS in the United States by 42% from 1996 to 1997 and by 20% from 1997 to 1998. Those living with HIV/AIDS on HAART felt stronger and healthier;

some even went back to work. With such remarkable results, HAART should be given to every HIV/AIDS patient. But the complications attendant to the medications warrant selective management.

In July 1996, a panel of experts assembled by the International AIDS Society issued a set of recommendations to doctors and other health care providers for antiretroviral therapy. The panel recommended treatment with three drugs—two NRTIs with one PI or one NRTI, one NNRTI, and a PI. This HAART was to be given to patients with (1) AIDS-defining illness, (2) CD4 count less than 500 cells/ml, particularly less than 350 cells/ml, or (3) viral load more than 30,000 copies/ml. Therapy was to be considered when viral load was above 10,000 copies/ml, particularly in the presence of other illnesses. The panel later recommended therapy for all patients with viral load above 10,000 copies/ml irrespective of CD4 count and the presence of other illnesses (Carpenter et al, 1997).

The medical treatment of HIV/AIDS is done with the biology of HIV pathogenesis in mind. Recall from the last chapter that HIV infection and pathogenesis of AIDS are nothing more than the destruction of human immune system by HIV so that the victim is left vulnerable to opportunistic infections. The purpose of antiretroviral therapy, therefore, is to reduce the number of viruses (viral load) in the patients as much as possible. Once the viral load is reduced, preferably to undetectable levels, the body can then regenerate immune cells to increase the CD4 count. And the increased CD4 level would allow the body to ward off infections by other organisms, thereby delaying the onset of opportunistic infections. Thus the ideal antiretroviral therapy would involve drugs powerful enough to eradicate HIV from the body, but not be toxic to the patient, and be reasonably priced to be affordable by all HIV/AIDS patients. Ultimately, the patient would have a better quality of life.

The initial success with HAART led to the suggestion that HIV disease could be cured; that is, as long as viral load remained undetectable and the patient was doing well clinically, a cure had been achieved. But in many patients viral load started going back up and CD4 count going down after being on HAART for a period of time. This was due to the fact that some viruses remained latent for years inside the human cells, then they slowly reproduced. Recall that these medications work to disrupt the reproductive cycle of HIV, so they are ineffective if the virus is not multiplying. The end result is the production of viruses that were resistant to the drugs. This phenomenon necessitated revision of HAART recommendations.

Subsequently, the United States Department of Health and Human Services (DHHS) issued a set of more flexible guidelines for antiretroviral therapy. The guidelines were based on the stage of the disease (see table 4.2). The DHHS guidelines are similar to the International AIDS Society recommendations. Treatment should be offered to patients with symptoms, those who have low CD4 count (less than 350 cells/ml), or those with very high viral load (100,000 copies/ml). For asymptomatic patients, treatment is recommended for those with CD4 count below 500 cell/ml or viral load greater than 20,000 copies/ml.

Table 4.2   Recommendations for the Intiation of Antiretroviral Therapy in Chronically HIV Infected Patients

CLINICAL CATEGORY	CD4 COUNT AND VIRAL LOAD	RECOMMENDATION
Symptomatic (fever, thrush, opportunistic infection)	Any value	Treat
Asymptomatic	CD4 count < 500 cells/ml or viral load > 20,000 copies/ml	Treatment should be offered; recommendation is based on disease advancement and patient's willingness to adhere to chronic therapy
Asymptomatic	CD4 > 500 cells/ml or viral load < 20,000 copies/ml	Treatment may be delayed or started based on discussion between provider and patient

SOURCE: United States Department of Health and Human Services

The decision to offer treatment is based on disease stage and willingness of the patient to comply with long-term therapy. For asymptomatic patients with CD4 count of more than 500 cells/ ml and viral load less than 20,000 copies/ml, health care providers would decide to delay treatment or start it based on individual patient characteristics and circumstances. However, many experts would delay therapy and observe the patient with those kinds of numbers. The reason for delaying therapy in these asymptomatic patients is that they generally feel well, and they may start feeling ill just because they are on treatment due to toxic side effects of the medications (Jacobson & Hicks, 2000).

Blood testing is a paramount concomitant of drug treatment of HIV/AIDS. Indeed diagnosis of HIV infection is done first with blood testing that is started with the HIV antibody test (initial ELISA test, followed by Western Blot confirmation test). Once positive antibody test is established, the next test to be performed is the CD4 count to determine how much damage the virus has done to the immune system. Then a viral load test is performed to determine the number of viruses in the body. Once therapy is commenced, the CD4 count and viral load levels are determined periodically to monitor the patient's progress.

Just as CD4 count and viral load are a marker of disease progression, they are a marker of how well the medications are working. The clinician should ideally see patients once a month after initiation of the medical therapy. The clinician assesses the patient's progress based on history taking, physical examination, and blood testing. Also how the patient is tolerating the medications is discussed during these visits. If CD4 count and viral load worsen after a period of improvement on medication, it indicates either the virus has become resistant to the medications or the patient might not be taking the medications as directed, or both. Indeed, non-compliance with therapy, not taking the medication as prescribed, often allows the virus to undergo mutation to resistant virus. When a patient who is doing well on medication starts getting worse, the clinician has to figure out why the patient is getting worse. If the reason for the drug failure is resistance, then alternative medications may be explored. However, if the failure is due to non-compliance with medication, then the clinician needs to find ways to effect better compliance.

Drug resistance

Drug resistance in HIV therapy is based on the genetic make-up of the virus. Like other RNA viruses, HIV lacks the ability DNA viruses have to maintain its genetic composition during the process of replication (making new copies of itself). Because of this characteristic, HIV may produce new strains containing drug resistant mutations. This could occur before antiretroviral medications are introduced (Hirsch et al, 1998). A mutant virus has the ability to elude the human immune system's ability to destroy it and also the action of medications.

Once a patient with a mutant HIV strain takes an antiretroviral medication, that strain continues to reproduce itself unaffected by the medication. The virus may have a single or multiple mutations in its genome. For some medications in the NRTI and NNRTI classes, a single mutation can cause drug resistance. For some other medications, especially from the PI class, drug resistance may require multiple mutations (Hirsch et al, 1998).

If a patient with drug resistant virus happens to transmit HIV to another person, the newly infected patient cannot be treated with the medications to which the virus is resistant in the original patient. Furthermore, there is the phenomenon of cross-resistance. Here a mutation that causes resistance to a particular antiretroviral medication may cause resistance to other drugs in the same class.

Drug resistance is a major problem for clinicians and patients alike in the management of HIV/AIDS. Even more problematic is the spread of drug resistant viruses. For example, drug resistant HIV has been isolated in some parts of Africa where the use of antiretroviral medications is not widespread. Patients who might have drug resistant viruses need to undergo blood testing to figure out the possible combination of antiretroviral medications appropriate for them.

Blood testing for drug resistance employs two methods— genotypic and phenotypic assays. Genotypic assays analyse reverse transcriptase and protease gene sequences of HIV fragments for mutants to test for resistance to specific drugs. In phenotypic assays, cells are infected with the patient's virus and tested with different drugs to determine the amount needed to inhibit viral growth (Jacobson and Hick, 2000). Both methods have their problems and shortcomings, but the biggest problem is cost. The tests are so expensive that clinicians do not routinely utilize them. Besides, only specialized laboratories can perform the assays.

Most clinicians base their decision on why a patient's clinical status is worsening on empirical evidence. If a drug that worked in the past does not seem to be working anymore, it could be due to drug resistance, patient non-compliance, or both. The usual approach is to try a new combination of medications, and emphasize to the patient the critical need for compliance with the therapy.

Non-compliance with therapy.

Compliance with medications, taking them exactly as directed, is of paramount importance in therapeutic outcome. "As directed" involves many aspects of taking a medication—how many pills, how many times a day; whether to take on empty stomach or with food; time difference between doses; and perhaps most importantly, making sure to take all the medication until it's all gone. Also to be considered is which drugs cannot be taken with which. It is not easy to follow directions on medication taking completely, particularly when multiple medications have to be taken, each having some unpleasant side effects. The difficulties attendant to taking medicine as directed often leads to non-compliance.

Medication non-compliance has been defined as the overuse, under-use, and misuse of medications (Cramer, 1995). The phenomenon has been part of medical history since the time of Hypocrates. Patients who have to take medicine for a long time or forever for such chronic conditions as hypertension, asthma, and diabetes often have difficulty complying with the therapy. This is because they often feel fine and either see no need to take the medicine or forget to do so when there is no pain or other symptom to remind them to take the medicine. It is estimated that on average only about 50% of all patients take medications as directed. The figure is even smaller, about 30%, when they have to take medicine for prophylaxis (taking the medicine to prevent the onset of a disease) or the medication is for long-term therapy (Haynes et al, 1996).

Medical management of HIV/AIDS is particularly challenging as far as compliance is concerned. HIV/AIDS patients have to contend with multiple regimens that keep changing, that involve strict schedules, timing of meal and fluid intake, and side effects such as nausea, vomiting, and diarrhoea. Some of the medications even cause new diseases that require a whole new set of medications. Non-compliance with antiretroviral medications, like most other medications, leads to poor therapeutic outcome and drug resistance.

Studies have shown that high levels of compliance with antiretroviral medications leads to decreased viral load, increased CD4 count, and decreased mortality. On the other hand, low compliance has the opposite and sometimes dramatic effect. For example, a decrease in compliance of 10% has been found to be associated with the doubling of viral load. The same 10% decrease was associated with 16% increase in mortality (Bartlett et al, 2000). Overall, it has been estimated that at least 95% compliance is required to decrease viral load to below a level of detection. When 90% compliance is achieved, only 37% of patients had viral load below detectable levels. However, only 28% of patients have been found to be able to achieve the requisite 95% or more level of compliance (Bartlett et al, 2000).

The problem of non-compliance has to be addressed by clinicians in order to improve therapeutic outcome and prevent emergence of drug resistant viruses. Patient education is the key; that is, the clinician should educate the patient about the critical importance of compliance, and possibly develop an individualized schedule for taking the medications. The clinician should try to ascertain the level of compliance by the patient at each visit; then try to suggest solutions to problems that caused any possible episodes of non-compliance (Jacobson & Hick, 2000). Patient education, of course, should take into consideration the patient's literacy level. It may be necessary to provide a detailed written instruction in a language the patient can understand. Of particular importance is education on how to deal with adverse side effects of the medications.

The potential for medication non-compliance (overuse, under-use, or misuse of medication) is much higher in countries where a doctor's written prescription is not required. This is the situation in many European and African countries. In many African countries, overuse and misuse of medication may be in the form of a recommendation by non-medical personnel such as a friend or relative. In this regard, medicine may be taken without diagnosis or for the wrong disease. Sometimes medicine may be taken without a specific ailment; it is taken to "feel better". Such medicines are often not taken properly. Under-use may be from the sharing of medicine prescribed for a particular person with friends or family members. Also, the patient may stop taking the medicine as soon as symptoms subside in order to save some of it for a "rainy day". In other situations, the patient simply cannot afford to buy the full amount of the prescription and may buy the partial amount that can be paid for. All these problems can lead to potential side effects and the emergence of drug resistance.

Obviously, antiretroviral medications are much more difficult to comply with in many of these countries when multiple medications are to be taken, when they have complicated schedule and serious side effects. The potential for misuse or under-use is high in light of the fact that these medicines are so expensive. And there may be difficulty in giving detailed written instructions to patients if the clinician's language is different from the patient's. Finally, there may not be the personnel or time to provide the necessary education to improve compliance.

Side effects of antiretroviral therapy.

That antiretroviral medications do have side effects should be no surprise to anyone because practically every medication has some side effects. The problem with antiretroviral medications is that side effects tend to be more numerous and often more incapacitating; some of them are even fatal. The complications tend to be serious because of the need for combination therapy. Even more problematic is that some of the antiretroviral medications cause new diseases that have to be treated with a new set of medications. And some of the other medications may interact with the antiretroviral medications to cause a whole new set of diseases. It can become a matter of "chasing your tail"; it can be very expensive...and frustrating indeed.

Severe side effects were noticed with the very first antiretroviral medication used to treat HIV/AIDS. Retrovir (AZT), an NRTI, was the first antiretroviral medication approved. Its side effects included abdominal pain, nausea, vomiting, anorexia (lack of appetite), headache, and neuropathy (pain and numbness in the extremities). Most of these side effects were what I call "nuisance symptoms"; that is, they were not life threatening. The symptoms were treated relatively simply, and the patients usually continued taking the medication. But there were rare cases of bone marrow toxicity that caused life threatening anaemia, often requiring blood transfusion.

The next NRTIs to be approved were Didanosine (ddI) and Zalcitabine (ddC). They did not have as many side effects as AZT, but they caused a more severe neuropathy and pancreatitis. The succeeding NRTIs had similar side effects to the earlier ones. And *Abacavir*, one of the newest NRTIs, can cause potentially fatal hypersensitivity reactions that are characterized by fever, rash, nausea, vomiting, and malaise (Jacobson & Hick, 2000). Indeed, hypersensitivity reactions can occur with any of the antiretroviral medications and other drugs used to treat HIV-related complications. The management of pancreatitis and hypersensitivity is the stopping of the offending medications.

All the NRTIs can cause mitochondrial dysfunction. *Mitochondria* are cell organelles that are involved in the production of *Adenosine Triphosphate* (ATP), which is a source of energy for various human tissues. The mitochondrial dysfunction caused by NRTIs reduces the amount of ATP. When this reduction occurs, tissues which require a lot of energy such as those of the liver, pancreas, heart, kidneys, and the nervous system, may be damaged (Chen et al, 1991). But the most serious effect of NRTIs on mitochondria is the production of lactic acidosis that is potentially fatal. Lactic acidosis usually occurs after long use of NRTIs. The symptoms of lactic acidosis include nausea, vomiting, abdominal pain, and hyperventilation. Treatment of lactic acidosis is the stopping of NRTIs (Brinkman et al, 1999).

As stated earlier, some side effects of antiretroviral therapy produced nuisance symptoms. As more antiretroviral medications were added to the anti-HIV armamentarium, more side effects, some resulting in other chronic syndromes, started to emerge. These chronic syndromes are mostly due to the PIs. The following are some of the chronic conditions associated with HAART.

1.   Osteopenia/Osteoporosis. Recent studies have found a higher incidence of osteopenia and osteoporosis (low bone mineral density) in people on PIs. The damage to bone by therapeutic toxicity of HAART has been associated with avascular necrosis of the hip and compression fractures of the lumbar spine (Tebas etal, 2000). Fractures are particularly likely in patients with AIDS wasting syndrome. Again when patients on PIs who developed osteopenia were switched to PI-sparing regimens, their low bone mineral density improved.

2.   Cardiovascular complications. There is a definite association between HAART and increased serum cholesterol and triglyceride levels. Since high serum levels of these lipids are a known risk factor for coronary heart disease, the issue of increased incidence of heart attacks in people on HAART has been raised. Though studies have demonstrated no increased incidence of heart attack among people on HAART, it seems to be just a matter of time. As people live longer on HAART, the risk of cardiovascularcomplications will increase because of hyperlipidemia. What is evident now is increased risk of hypertension (high blood pressure). Studies have demonstrated an association between hypertension and HAART therapy. The increased risk for hypertension in HAART patients is likely due to hyperlipidemia (Johnson et al, 2000).

3.   Sexual dysfunction. Sexual dysfunction in HIV/AIDS patients

has been known for some time. The nature of a chronic debilitating illness often causes sexual dysfunction. In addition to the disease itself, depression that often accompanies the disease may cause sexual dysfunction. However, recent evidence has suggested an association between PI therapy and sexual dysfunction (Colson et al, 2000).

4. Lipodystrophy syndrome. Perhaps the most serious and complicated of the chronic illnesses resulting from HAART is lipodystrophy syndrome. This is often characterized by abdominal obesity ("protease paunch"), peripheral fat wasting ("AIDS face"), build up of inter-scapular fat ("buffalo hump"), hyperlipidemia, and insulin resistance (Carr et al, 1998; Jacobson & Hick, 2000). A rare condition that occurs as part of the lipodystrophy syndrome is lipomas (benign fatty tumours). Lipomastosis is characterized by non-tender tumours on the upper trunk, neck, back of the head, and arms (Meza & Verghese, 1999).

The most serious chronic conditions of the lipodystrophy syndrome are hyperlipidemia and insulin resistance. As stated earlier, high serum cholesterol and triglyceride levels are a long-term risk for heart attacks and other cardiovascular complications. Insulin resistance leads to diabetes in these patients. And diabetes is risk factor for cardiovascular disease. Therefore, patients on HAART who develop hyperlipidemia and diabetes have to be treated lest they die from lypodystrophy complications instead of AIDS. And this phenomenon has been reported. Diabetes is particularly bad because of its numerous complications that include blindness, heart failure, kidney failure, peripheral vascular disease that could lead to lower extremity amputations, and sexual dysfunction in males.

Studies have shown that when patients with lipodystrophy were switched from PIs to NNRTIs, their metabolic abnormalities might return to normal in three months and their body composition after one year (Jacobson & Hick, 2000). Dietary modification and exercise help in decreasing truncal and total body fat. In addition to changing antiretroviral medications and employing dietary changes and exercise, treating hyperlipidemia and diabetes is warranted.

Hyperlipidemia has been treated with a variety of medications, but the class of drugs called statins are the most effective in lowering both cholesterol and triglyceride levels (Jacobson & Hicks, 2000). However, all PIs are known to cause damage to the liver; and the toxicity of the liver and muscle pain are side effects of the statins. HAART-induced diabetes is treated with insulin-sensitising medications such as Metformin. And muscle wasting has been treated with human growth hormone (hGH) with limited results; it has also been treated with testosterone. All these medications have a tendency to affect the liver adversely. Furthermore, hGH is very expensive and has some other bad side effects. Metformin and the other insulin-sensitising medications are also quite expensive.

From the discussion on antiretroviral therapy so far, it is obvious that management of HIV/AIDS with antiretroviral medications is a daunting task indeed. It requires a long-term, perhaps life-long, commitment to complex regimens. These regimens involve taking many pills two or three times a day, food and fluid modifications, medication toxicities, and having to deal with drug-induced new diseases. All these have the potential to change the patient physically (as in lipodystrophy syndrome) and the patient's lifestyle. Then the patient might not take the medicines as directed because of these problems. And non-compliance with medications may lead to the emergence of drug resistant viruses. In many situations, these problems lead patients and their doctors to consider modification of the drug regimen. What can they do when there is a need to change a particular regimen?

The reason for considering changing medication regimens are usually to (1) improve compliance by reducing pill burden, food requirements, and dosing frequency, (2) reduce the potential for drug-drug interactions, (3) manage drug toxicities, and (4) establish another treatment plan with a new class or combination of drugs. The new regimen should ideally be able to keep viral load down, CD4 count up, have few (tolerable) toxic effects, and improve quality of life (Moyles, 2000).

Switching antiretroviral medications usually means switching from PI containing to PI-sparing regimens. This is because most of the problematic issues involve the protease inhibitors. However, the NRTIs also have serious problems particularly in terms of toxicity and drug resistant viruses. That leaves the NNRTIs as the only rescue class of antiretroviral medications. Recall that of the 16 drugs approved as anti-HIV/AIDS therapy by the end of the year 2000, only three were in that class. This is rather limited in terms of choice; besides, the NNRTIs are not problem free either. Therefore, other approaches are being explored.

Some of the approaches suggested include delaying initiation of therapy, using less intensive therapy, and employing pulse therapy or repeated therapy interruption (Moyles, 2000). This means the "hit them early, hit them hard" and HAART approaches are falling out of favour. The new approach is aimed at making therapy simpler and less expensive. "The simpler, the better" is an adage HIV/AIDS researchers are looking at keenly.

Simplification of medication regimen is most critically needed in terms of pill burden for patients. Studies have shown that there is better compliance when patients take one or two medicines once or twice a day than multiple medications three or more times a day. In this regard, the studies found that a lower percentage of patients on regimens with higher pill burden achieved viral load below detectable levels (Bartlett et al, 2000). Obviously, patients with the higher pill burden took the medicine as directed less often, hence their lower rate of viral suppression. Since non-compliance is a potential cause of drug resistance, addressing the issue of high pill burden is very important. Therefore, the need for research into development of simpler antiretroviral medications is rather obvious. Therefore recent development whereby two or more of the antiretroviral medications are combined into one pill to be taken once or twice a day is welcome news indeed.

With all the problems attendant to antiretroviral medications, the US Department of Health and Human Services (DHHS) issued another set of recommendations for the initiation of antiretroviral therapy in 2001. By the new guidelines, the previous recommendations for those with symptomatic disease would still apply. For asymptomatic patients the new guidelines suggest treatment be delayed until CD4 count is below 350 cells/ml or viral load is above 55,000 copies/ml. The guidelines were issued largely in recognition of (1) the increasing number of antiretroviral treatment-related side effects; (2) the realization that antiretroviral therapy alone is not likely to eradicate HIV infection, that patients might be on these medicines for a life time; and (3) the fact that non-compliance and resistance are major unresolved issues (Eron, 2001).

Management Of Opportunistictic Infections

I have often said in my speeches that HIV, the virus that causes AIDS, has not killed anyone yet. What it does is to destroy a person's immune system such that other organisms would cause the death associated with AIDS. Indeed, the presence of opportunistic infections is largely a prerequisite for the definition of AIDS. Many of the organisms associated with AIDS usually do not cause serious disease in people with intact immune system. With the destruction of the immune system in AIDS, these organisms now have "the opportunity" to cause disease and ultimate death. Therefore, the diseases these otherwise harmless organisms cause are termed *opportunistic infections*. Because AIDS is the result of total immune destruction, AIDS patients may develop opportunistic infections with organisms from all major microbial groups; some examples follow:

(1). Protozoa: *pneumocystis carinii*, toxoplasma, cryptosporidium, giardia, amoeba.

(2). Fungi: candida, cryptococcus, coccidioiodomycosis

(3). Viruses: cytomegalovirus (CMV), Epstein-Barr virus (EBV), herpes simplex, herpes zoster

(4). Bacteria: *Mycobacterium tuberculosis, Mycobacterium avium intracellulare,* salmonella

Since opportunistic infections are related to weakened immune system, there is increased incidence of these infections at low CD4 counts. In general, patients with CD4 counts at 500 cells/ml or above do not get opportunistic infections, and those with 200 cell/ml or below are at a very high risk of developing them. Once acquired, these opportunistic infections are difficult to treat; there are not many effective and safe anti-microbial medications to cure these infections. Therefore, it is more appropriate to prevent than to treat.

Ideally opportunistic infections should be prevented by keeping the CD4 count above 200 cells/mm, preferably above 500 cells/mm. As stated earlier, the use of HAART has dramatically reduced death rates from opportunistic infections among American and European patients. However, the vast majority of HIV/AIDS patients worldwide do not have access to the antiretroviral medications. Even in the United States, poor people with HIV/ AIDS who have limited access to HAART and general medical care continue to have high mortality rates from opportunistic infections. Furthermore, the problems with side effects, drug resistance, and drug-induced metabolic diseases make HAART no more the best approach to preventing opportunistic infections.

Rather simple measure such as avoidance of uncooked or under cooked foods, unpasteurized dairy products, unfiltered or un-boiled water, and unwashed salad ingredients and fruits can help prevent exposure to many of these organisms. Also, HIV/

AIDS patients with low CD4 count should avoid contact with people who may be harbouring infections and other potentially communicable diseases. In addition to the above measures, prophylactic medications should be taken when CD4 count is below 200 cells/mm. *Prophylaxis* is the taking of medication to prevent the occurrence of a particular disease.

For opportunistic infection prophylaxis, that for *pneumocystis carinii* (PCP), *toxoplasmosis*, *Mycobacteria avium complex* (MAC), and candidiasis is the most often undertaken. Medicines used to treat the actual disease are taken prophylactically, often in lower doses than what is used to treat the actual disease. Obviously the taking of prophylactic medications in addition to antiretroviral medications adds to the pill burden and compounds drug side effects. Furthermore, some of these prophylactic medications are very expensive. Therefore, when CD4 count goes up significantly and stays up for a period of time, prophylactic medication might be discontinued (Jacobson & Hicks, 2000).

REFERENCES

1. Bartlett, J. et al (2000). Correlation between antiretroviral pill burden and durability of virologic responses: a systematic overview. In *Abstracts of XIII International AIDS Conference July 9-14, 2000*; Durban, South Africa. Abstract Th Pe B4998

2. Brinkman, K. et al (1998). Adverse effects of reverse transcriptase inhibitors Mitochondrial toxicity as common pathway. *AIDS*; 12: 1735-1744.

3. Brinkman, K. et al (1999). Mitochondrial toxicity induced by nucleoside analogue reverse transcriptase inhibitors is a key factor in the pathogenesis of antiviral therapy-related lipodystrophy. *Lancet*;

354:1112-1115.

4. Carr, A. et al (1998). A syndrome of peripheral lipodystrophy, hyperlipidemia, and insulin resistance in patients receiving HIV protease inhibitors. *AIDS*; 12: F51-F58.

5. Chen, C. et al (1991). Effect of anti-human immunodeficiency virus nucleoside analogues on mitochondrial DNA and its implications for delayed toxicity. *Molec Pharmcol*; 39:625-628.

6. Colson, A. et al (2000). Sexual dysfunction in protease inhibitor recipients. In: *Program and Abstracts of 7th Conference on Retrovirus and Opportunistic Infections, January 30-February 2, 2000;* San Francisco, Calif. Abstract 63.

7. Cramer, J.A. (1995). Partial medication compliance: the enigma in medical outcomes. *American Journal of Managed Care*; I (2): 167-174.

8. D'Souza, M. (2000). Current evidence and future directions for targeting HIV entry: therapeutic and prophylactic strategies. *Journal of American Medical Assoc*; 284(2) 215222.

9. Eron, Jr, J.J. (2001). Initial therapy: when to start, what to start with. *Selected Summaries from the 8th Conference on Retroviruses and Opportunistic infections, February 4-8, 2001,* Chicago, IL; p. 1-11.

10. Grinspoon, S. et al (1998). Effects of androgen administration in men with AIDS wasting syndrome: a randomised, double blind, placebo controlled trial. *Ann Intern Med*; 129: 18-26.

11. Haynes, R.B. et al (1996). Systematic review of randomised trials of intervention to assist patients to follow prescription for medications. *Lancet*; 348: 383-386.

12. Henderson, C.W. (2000). Interleukin-2 treatment plus antiretroviral therapy significantly increases CD4 cell count. *AIDS Weekly*, July 24, 2000; 5-8.

13. Hirsch, M. et al (1998). Antiretroviral drug resistance testing in adults with HIV infection. *Journal American Medical Assoc*, 279: 1984-1991.

14. Jacobson, M.A. and Hicks, M.L. (2000). *HIV Treatment: A Primer for Primary Care Clinicians;* Chicago: Meniscus.

15. Lands, L. (2000). Beyond eradication...*POZ*, 3/200; 62-63.

16. Lederman, M.M. and Valdez, H. (2000). Immune restoration with antiretroviral therapies: Implications for clinical management. *Journal American Medical Assoc*, 284 (2); 21 5222.

17. Johnson, D.L. et al (2000). Hypertension in HIV patients with metabolic dysfunction. In: *Program and Abstracts of 7th Conference on Retroviruses and Opportunistic Infections, January 30-February 2, 2000*; San Francisco,Calif. Abstract 36.

18. Lo, J.C. et al (1998). "Buffalo hump" in men with HIV-1 infection. *Lancet*, 351; 867-870.

19. Meza, A.D. and Verghese, A. (1999). Upper body lipomas in an HIV infected man. *Hospital Practice*, April 15, 1999; 130-135.

20. Moyle, G. (2000). Controversies in antiretroviral management: The need for simpler, cheaper, and safer therapy. *Conference Summaries from the XIII International AIDS Conference, July 9-14, 2000*, Durban, South Africa.

21. Moyle, G. (2000). Does therapy simplification always simplify therapy? *Selected Summaries from the 40th Inter-science Conference on Antimicrobial Agents & Chemotherapy, September 17-20, 2000*, Toronto, Ontario, Canada.

22. Silva M. et al (1998). The effect of protease inhibitors on weight and body composition in HIV-infected patients. *AIDS*, 12; 1645-1651.

23. Tebas, P. et al (2000). Accelerated bone mineral loss in HIV-infected patients receiving antiretroviral therapy. *AIDS*, 14; F63-F67.

24. Van der Horst, C and Wohl, D.A. (2000). Opportunistic infections in the era of HAART. *Conference Summaries from the XIII International AIDS Conference, July 9-14, 2000*, Durban, South Africa.

CHAPTER FIVE

AIDS IN AFRICA

The expression "Africa is burning" was first used by AIDS activists at the conclusion of the 12th International AIDS Conference in Zurich, Switzerland, in 1998. According to the activists, Africa was burning because it had been ignored for so long. Whereas HIV/AIDS patients in the developed world were living longer and healthier lives because of powerful antiretroviral medications, their counterparts in Africa were dying because of a lack of access to these life-saving drugs. Not only were these medications prohibitively expensive, international trade laws prevented companies in Africa from developing cheaper generic equivalents of those drugs. The multinational drug companies of the West were accused of genocide against Africans.

The shouting of "Africa is burning" at the conclusion of the 12th International AIDS Conference was in protest of the unacceptable situation of nonavailability of antiretroviral medications in Africa. Activists demanded that the drug companies should stop ignoring Africa and make the drugs available and affordable there. But it is not just the drug companies that had ignored Africa regarding the AIDS epidemic. International agencies, governments of the developed world, and African governments had not done what they should have to control the epidemic in Africa. It is not just the lack of access to expensive medications; until recently, Africa had virtually been ignored since the beginning of the epidemic.

Very early during the epidemic, there was speculation that Africa was a hopeless case as far as the AIDS epidemic was concerned, and nothing much could be done about the situation there. In March 1987, a group of AIDS experts, under the auspices of UNICEF, met at the Tufts University European Center in Talloires, France, to discuss AIDS and development. One of the consensus statements at the end of the meeting was:

> The idea that somehow Africa might already be lost to AIDS...is a preposterous idea. Even in African countries where the infection is already real and widespread, it still affects only small numbers relative to the whole population. The idea that a whole generation in some African countries should be written off is acceptable neither in human nor developmental terms (Duh, 1991; p. 54).

At the time this statement was issued in 1987, the WHO had received only about 50,000 reported cases of AIDS from about 40 countries in Africa. And only five or six countries had cases anywhere near what could be considered hopeless. It is true that there were no reported cases of AIDS in many African countries at that time, and in the countries where cases had been identified, the epidemic was not at a level of hopelessness. But the potential existed for the epidemic to spread and worsen to the point of hopelessness. This is because the political, economic, and health infrastructure in most African countries was not adequate to control even a small epidemic. These countries depended on external sources for help. And some of these external sources were using excuses to ignore Africa.

One of the reasons for the notion that Africa should be written off was the perception that AIDS in Africa was different from AIDS in other countries. This perception was based on the fact that AIDS in Africa affected males and females about equally, whereas in other parts of the world it was a predominantly male disease. In the consensus statement at the UNICEF conference cited above was the following statement. The statement was entitled, "Dangerous Misconception":

> There is a widespread myth that AIDS in Africa, and the way it is transmitted, is somehow different from AIDS in developed countries, and therefore causes some planetary danger. African AIDS is transmitted in exactly the same way as AIDS in other societies. It does not jump out of trees at visiting tourists or businessmen. We are talking sex and blood transmission (Duh, 1991; p. 53).

So with the perception that African AIDS was different, many people outside the continent regarded Africa as a lost cause. They perceived that millions of Africans had been infected by HIV and were dying from AIDS. And the kind of AIDS they were dying from was different from that of other parts of the world. Parts of the continent were so ravaged by AIDS that nothing much could be done about it.

As stated earlier, millions of people were *not* dying from AIDS in Africa by 1987. In addition to the United Nations, as exemplified by the UNICEF statement above, others from Africa took exception to the fact that millions were dying. Indeed, the president of Uganda stated in a television interview in 1985 that AIDS did not exist in his country. AIDS was a disease of homosexuals and intravenous drug users, and there were no homosexuals or drug users in Uganda. Dr. Konotey-Ahulu, a Ghanaian physician, was another person who wrote about his discontent with the idea that millions of Africans were dying from AIDS.

In a 1987 article in the British medical journal *Lancet*, Konotey-Ahulu, then of Cromwell Hospital in London, challenged the idea. He had travelled through 15 sub-Saharan African countries to assess the AIDS situation there. He took particular exception to the labelling of the whole continent. He stated that there were 51 countries in Africa, and only five or six of them had major problems with AIDS. Why were the remaining countries being so labelled? He expressed frustration at reports of rampant deaths from AIDS. "If tens of thousands are dying from AIDS (and Africans do not cremate their dead), where are the graves" (Konotey-Ahulu, 1987; p. 207).

In an earlier book (Duh, 1991), I expressed my agreement with the UNICEF statement and Konotey-Ahulu's article. I agreed that AIDS in Africa was no different, and it was not killing millions of people. By August 1990, a total of 70,724 cases of AIDS had been reported to the WHO from 45 African countries. I asserted that even if one assumed that the number represented only one-tenth of actual cases, AIDS still did not kill that many people. Other diseases were more devastating than AIDS. For example, malaria killed about a million people, and measles, tuberculosis, and diarrhoeal diseases killed millions more. I concluded: "AIDS is not killing millions of African now, *but it has the potential to do just that if the world permits* (Duh, 1991; p. 55). (Italics added). I am afraid the world did permit, and by the end of the year 2000 AIDS had killed more than 17 million Africans! That means in just 10 years, we went from fewer than 100,000 deaths to more than 17 millions deaths; and millions more were living with the condition on the continent.

Epidemiology Of HIV/AIDS In Africa

I consider the epidemiology of HIV/AIDS in Africa a matter of "What went wrong?" The epidemic started slowly on the continent, spread rather slowly initially, and then exploded to involve almost the whole continent. Many, if not most, countries in Africa were spared the initial onslaught of the epidemic (see Table 5. 1). But by the year 2000 almost every country, big and small, rich and poor, was being badly affected (see table 5.2). However, the distribution of HIV/AIDS cases in Africa has been uneven. Also, the distribution within countries has been uneven. The question is what went wrong? Why was the epidemic not controlled when the number of cases was small, when only a few countries were affected? Why did the epidemic spread so fast in Africa at a time when it was slowing down in the West? Why is the largest majority of HIV/AIDS cases in the world occurring in Africa?

The first cases of AIDS in Africa were reported to the WHO in 1982. By August 31, 1990, 70,724 cases of AIDS had been reported to the WHO from 45 African countries (see Table 5.1). Those cases represented the cumulative total of cases since the disease was first recognized on the continent. Of the 45 countries, 24 had reported more than 100 cases, and 9 of those countries had reported more than 1,000 cases. Of the nine countries reporting more than 1,000 cases, only Ghana and the Cote d'Ivoire were in West Africa, with the rest being in Central and contagious East African countries. Furthermore, all the countries with more than 10 cases per 100,000 population were in Central and East Africa except Cote d'Ivoire (Duh, 1991).

Estimates of HIV infection in Africa in 1990 paralleled the number of reported cases of AIDS, with a ratio of about 3: 1. So if one assumed three cases of HIV infection for each case of full-blown AIDS, the possible number of people living HIV/AIDS in 1990 was fewer than 300,000. If one assumed that only 10% of cases were reported, then a maximum of about three million HIV/AIDS cases might have existed in Africa then. In other words, the epidemic of HIV/AIDS in Africa in 1990 was totally manageable. A decade later, the epidemic was a truly catastrophic one, getting close to uncontrollable in some countries.

As of the end of the year 2000, UNAIDS estimates 25.3 million cases of HIV/AIDS in Africa. By that number, Africa had 70% of adults and 80% of children living with HIV/AIDS in the world. In addition, 17 million Africans had died from AIDS since the beginning of the epidemic, representing 75% of the 21.8 million AIDS deaths worldwide. Unlike other regions where the majority

Table 5.1. Number of AIDS cases reported to the WHO from African Countries as of the end of August 1990

Country	Cumulative Number of Cases
Algeria	45
Angola	104
Benin	60
Botswana	67
Burkina Faso	906
Burundi	2,784
Cameroon	78
Cape Verde	32
Central African Republic	662
Chad	35
Comoros	2
Congo	1,940
Cote d'Ivoire	3,647
Equatorial Guinea	3
Ethiopia	437
Gabon	64
Gambia	81
Ghana	1,252
Guinea	125
Guinea Bissau	123
Kenya	9,139
Lesotho	11
Liberia	5
Madagascar	2
Malawi	7,160
Mali	178
Mauritania	16
Mauritius	5
Mozambique	120
Namibia	232
Niger	80
Nigeria	48
Reunion	49
Rwanda	2,867
Sao Tome	2
Senegal	307
Sierra Leone	21
South Africa	463
Swaziland	14
Tanzania	7,128
Togo	100
Uganda	12,444
Zaire	11,732
Zambia	3,000
Zimbabwe	3,134
Total	**70,724**

SOURCE: WHO Global Programme on AIDS

of HIV/AIDS cases were in males, 55% of those in Africa were female. Obviously, if more females were living with HIV/AIDS, then more females were dying from AIDS. Therefore, Africa had more children orphaned by AIDS than any other region in the world (UNAIDS, 2001).

And so it goes. A manageable epidemic has exploded in 10 years to pose a potential threat to the survival of a whole continent. More importantly, the epidemic does not seem to have lost its fire. Each day an estimated 11,000 people are infected with HIV in Africa; each day an estimated 6000 Africans die from AIDS (Brown, 2001). The newly infected are even more likely to be female than those living with the condition. In some African countries, the rate of new infections in teenage girls is five times higher than in teenage boys; and among young people in their early 20s, it is three times higher in women (UNAIDS, 2001a).

As stated earlier, only a few countries in Africa were affected by HIV/AIDS in a serious way by 1990, but 10 years later many countries were being threatened. Even more disturbing is the devastation of some countries which were not affected by 1990. In 1990, almost all the countries seriously affected were in Central and East Africa; countries in West and Southern Africa had relatively few cases, with North Africa hardly having any cases. By the year 2000, all the countries that were truly "burning" were in Southern Africa.

The top eight countries in Africa as far as the adult prevalence of HIV/AIDS is concerned are all in Southern Africa. In fact, these countries also have the highest rates in the world—at least 15% each. In these eight countries AIDS would kill about a third of today's 15-year olds in the next 10 years (UNAIDS, 2001a). In Botswana, an alarming 36% of adults had HIV/AIDS in a country of about 1.5 million population. The Republic of South Africa, with an estimated 4.7 million infected had the largest number of people living with HIV/AIDS in the world. Its adult prevalence was about 20%. Other countries in Southern Africa that were "burning" with rates above 20% are Swaziland (25%), Zimbabwe (25%), and Lesotho (23%) (See table 5.2).

West Africa remained relatively less affected with adult rates below 2% in some countries. Cote d'Ivoire was the only country in West Africa with a rate above 10%. However, Nigeria, the most populous country in Africa (with over 120 million people), with a rate of about 2% had about 2.7 million people living with HIV/AIDS. East Africa, once with the highest rates on the continent, in 2000 had rates above those in West Africa but below those in Southern Africa (see table 5.3).

The rates in North Africa were still quite low; they parallel those of the Middle East. Indeed, in categorizing the prevalence of HIV/AIDS in different regions of the world, UNAIDS puts North Africa and the Middle East in one category. In addition to prevalence, the main mode of transmission of HIV in North Africa parallels that of the Middle East. Thus, when one talks about HIV/AIDS in Africa, one is actually referring to the epidemic in sub-Saharan Africa. The expression "Africa is burning" should technically be "sub-Saharan Africa is burning."

The geographical distribution of HIV/AIDS in different African countries parallels that in other parts of the world; that is, most cases are in urban areas. But the spread to rural areas is very

Table 5.2. Estimated number of people living with HIV/AIDS in Africa as of end of 2000 by alphabeticanl order of countries

Country	Adults (15-49)	Women (15-49)	Children (0-14)	Total	Rate (%)
Algeria	*	*	*	11,000	0.07
Angola	150,000	82,000	7,900	160,000	2.87
Benin	67,000	37,000	3,000	70,000	2.45
Botswana	280,000	150,000	10,000	290,000	35.80
Burkina Faso	330,000	180,000	20,000	350,000	6.44
Burundi	340,000	190,000	19,000	360,000	11.32
Cameroon	520,000	290,000	22,000	540,000	7.32
Central Africa Rep	230,000	130,000	8,900	240,000	13.4
Chad	88,000	49,000	4,000	92,000	2.69
Comoros	*	*	*	400	0.12
Congo	82,000	45,000	4,000	86,000	6.43
Cote d'Ivoire	750,000	400,000	32,000	760,000	10.73
Dem. Rep Congo	1,110,000	60,000	53,000	1,110,000	5.07
Djibouti	35,000	19,000	1,500	35,000	11.75
Egypt	*	*	*	8,100	0.02
Equ Guinea	1,000	560	<100	1,100	0.51
Eritrea	*	*	*	49,000	2.87
Ethiopia	2,900,000	1,600,000	150,000	3,000,000	10.63
Gabon	22,000	12,000	780	23,000	4.16
Gambia	12,000	6,600	520	13,000	1.95
Ghana	330,000	180,000	14,000	340,000	4.60
Guinea	52,000	29,000	2,700	55,000	1.54
Guinea Bissau	13,000	7,300	560	14,000	2.50
Kenya	2,000,000	1,100,000	78,000	2100,000	13.95
Lesotho	240,000	130,000	8,200	240,000	23.57
Liberia	37,000	21,000	2,000	39,000	2.80
Libya	*	*	*	1,400	0.05
Madagascar	10,000	5,800	450	11,000	0.15
Malawi	760,000	420,000	40,000	800,000	15.96
Mali	97,000	53,000	5,000	102,000	2.03
Mauritania	6,300	3,500	280	6,6000	0.52
Mauritius	*	*	*	500	0.08
Morocco	*	*	*	5,000	0.03
Mozambique	1,100,000	630,000	52,000	1,200,000	13.22
Namibia	150,000	85,000	6,600	160,000	19.54
Niger	61,000	34,000	3,300	64,000	1.35
Nigeria	2,600,000	1,400,000	1,200,000	2,700,000	2.06
Reunion	*	*	*	*	*
Rwanda	370,000	210,000	22,000	400,000	11.21
Senegal	76,000	40,000	3,300	79,000	1.71
Seychelles	*	*	*	*	*
Sierra Leone	65,000	36,000	3,300	68,000	2.99
Somalia	*	*	*	*	*
South Africa	4,500,000	2,600,000	1,000,000	4,700,000	19.94
Sudan	*	*	*	*	*
Swaziland	120,000	67,000	3,800	130,000	25.25
Togo	120,000	66,000	6,300	130,000	5.98
Tunisia	*	*	*	2200	*
Uganda	770,000	420,000	50,000	82,000	8.30
Tanzania	1,200,000	670,000	59,000	1,300,000	8.09
Zambia	830,000	450,000	40,000	870,000	19.95
Zimbabwe	1,400,000	800,000	56,000	1,500,000	25.06

\# Refers to adult rate, based on adult population of 15-49 years old

Source: Joint UN Programme on HIV/AIDS (UNAIDS)

Table 5.3. Countries with more than 10% rate of estimated number of adults living with HIV/AIDS in Sub Saharan africa as end of 2000

Country	Adults	Total	Prevalence Rate (%) #
1. Botswana	280,000	290,000	35.80
2. Swaziland	1,200,000	1,300,00	25.25
3. Zimbabwe	1,400,000	1,500,000	25.06
4. Lesotho	230,000	240,000	23.57
5. Zambia	830,000	870,000	19.95
6. South Africa	4,500,000	4,700,000	19.94
7. Namibia	150,000	160,000	19.54
8. Malawi	760,000	800,000	15.96
9. Kenya	2,000,000	2,100,000	13.95
10. Cent Afr Rep	230,000	240,000	13.84
11. Mozambique	1,100,000	1,200,000	13.22
12. Djibouti	35,000	37,000	11.75
13. Burundi	340,000	360,000	11.32
14. Rwanda	370,000	400,000	11.21
15. Cote d'Ivoire	730,000	760,000	10.73
16. Ethiopia	2,900,000	3,000,000	10.63

\# Refers to adult rate, based upon adult population of 15-49 year olds.

SOURCE: Joint UN Programme on HIV/AIDS (UNAIDS).

real in many countries. Also, significantly high rates of HIV infection are found among commercial sex workers, patients attending STD clinics, women attending antenatal clinics, and hospitalized patients. These trends are driven by the fact that heterosexual transmission is the main mode of HIV transmission in Africa (UNAIDS, 2001b).

The heterosexual transmission is fueling the epidemic in Africa. When HIV is spread among a small population as it is among homosexuals, there could be a temporary cap on the number of people exposed. However, when transmission is between men and women, more people are immediately at risk (UNAIDS, 2001 b). So the epidemic worsens as more newly infected people join it each year than leave it through death. In this regard, 3.8 million people were newly infected in the year 2000, while 2.4 million died the same year. The good news is that the 3.8 million new cases in 2000 were slightly lower than the 4.0 million in 1999. This has been attributed to effective prevention programs in some countries. Secondly, with adult infection rates of more than 25% in some countries, there are fewer people to be infected (UNAIDS, 2001a).

The question of what went wrong with the HIV/AIDS epidemic in Africa can be simply answered by the fact that not enough was done to control the epidemic when it was more manageable. The other question is why it spread so fast. For example, the adult prevalence in South Africa was less than 1% by 1990 but increased 12.9% in 1998 and to 19.9% in 2000 (UNAIDS, 2001b). Similarly, the prevalence n Botswana was less than 1% by 190 but increased to a whopping 36% by 2000. The tragic fact is that in none of the most heavily affected countries has the spread been checked. Since it takes 7-10 years from HIV diagnosis to death, almost all 25.3 million HIV/AIDS patients in Africa will die by the 2010 . . . unless a medical miracle occurs (Brown, 2001).

The devastation of HIV/AIDS among Africans has led some people to speculate that the condition is different in Africa, or there is something biologically different about Africans, which makes them more susceptible to the virus. In reference to the latter, the speculation is in regard to black people in general. This suggestion is made because of the disproportionately high prevalence among black Americans, Caribbean blacks, and African blacks. Then there is the suggestion that HIV does not cause AIDS at all. Those who hold that view, the so-called AIDS dissidents, claim that HIV does not cause AIDS; they contend that poverty is what causes AIDS. Black people everywhere suffer disproportionately from AIDS because black people suffer disproportionately from poverty.

That AIDS in Africa is different was a speculation earlier in the epidemic. Those who held this view pointed to the fact that there was an almost 1:1 ratio of male to female in Africa, whereas AIDS was a predominantly male disease in other parts of the world. Also African AIDS patients presented with a different clinical manifestation from those in Europe and the Americas.

Transmission Of HIV In Africa

As stated earlier, there are four general means of HIV transmission—sexually, needle sharing (in IV drug use), blood and blood products, and mother to child parentally and through breast-feeding. These are the same means of transmission in Africa except IV drug use is not very common. Although homosexual activity predominates in other parts of the world, heterosexual activity is the predominant sexual means of transmission in Africa. Obviously, heterosexual transmission necessarily results in the sharing of the virus between men and women, so the ratio of 1:1 should not be a surprise. However, blood transfusion and medical injections play a role in that ratio.

Because of technical and logistical problems, screening of transfusion blood for HIV was inadequate in many African countries. Thus, transfusion-associated HIV transmission continued in these countries well into the 1990s, whereas it was very rare elsewhere. Malnutrition and some endemic diseases such as malaria and sickle cell disease are a significant contributing factor to anaemia that would require blood transfusion. Also, blood transfusion is often required during childbirth. Young adults are the most likely to donate blood, and they have the highest HIV prevalence rates. So blood transfusion has been a significant contributor to the explosion of HIV/AIDS in Africa (Duh, 1991).

Medical injections is another way of transferring blood from one person to another. There is a widespread belief in many African countries that injected medication is more effective than oral medication. Patients (and parents of pediatric patients) often request injections if they are given oral medication at clinics and hospitals (Duh, 1991). The use of medical injections in many African countries is not limited to clinics and hospitals. Private individuals, particularly in rural areas, may keep some medication and injecting equipment at home to give injections to town folk. Also, some freestanding pharmacies and drug stores give injections.

In many cases, the private individuals and pharmacy personnel are inadequately trained in aseptic technique; there may be no facilities for adequate sterilization of needles and syringes. Even the clinics and hospitals may not perform adequate sterilization of injecting equipment. And the reuse of disposable needles and syringes is not uncommon. Many of these facilities do not have enough needles and syringes, so they do their best to clean disposable equipment for reuse. This process of using non-sterile needles and syringes is similar to needle (and blood) sharing among IV drug users, a process I refer to as *institutional needle sharing* (Duh, 1991). Again, medical injections are universal for males and females.

Perinatal transmission of HIV has persisted in Africa mainly because of the unavailability of antiretroviral medication for pregnant women. In most African countries, neither the government nor individuals can afford these drugs. Furthermore, because many pregnant women do not get routine prenatal care at hospitals and clinics, they would not be tested for HIV even if medicines were available to them. But in South Africa, it appears that the government deliberately did not make the drugs available because of President Mbeki's belief that HIV did not cause AIDS. Also breast-feeding is extremely prevalent in many African countries. It does contribute to mother-to-child transmission, especially if the mother does not know she is infected.

Clinical Manifestations Of AIDS In Africa

The clinical manifestations of AIDS described in Chapter Three of this book apply to African AIDS patients. They get certain types of cancers and opportunistic infections as do AIDS patients elsewhere. However, dermatological and gastro-intestinal problems are more common among Africans, whereas generalized lymphadenopathy and pulmonary problems are more common among American and European AIDS patients. The most common opportunistic infections among African AIDS patients are oral candidiasis, cryptococcal meningitis, cryptosporidiosis, and mycobacteria. In America and Europe, *pneumocystis carinii* pneumonia is the predominant opportunistic infection (Duh, 1991).

The clinical manifestations described above are displayed by native Africans and Europeans living in Africa. For example, Belgians living in Zaire (now the Democratic Republic of Congo), Rwanda, and Burundi were found in a study to have clinical manifestations akin to "African AIDS", not "European AIDS." There was also close to 1:1 ratio of male to female of HIV prevalence among these Belgians. The significant thing about this study was that the Belgians had been involved in or subjected to the same practices as native Africans. That is, they had had multiple heterosexual contact with native Africans, received blood transfusions, and been given numerous medical injections (Bonneaux, 1988).

The differences in clinical manifestations are not an indication of different kinds of AIDS. They are a reflection of an association between endemic diseases and AIDS. The basic definition of AIDS is the destruction of the body's immune system such that a person becomes subjected to common and unusual diseases. It makes sense then that a person with AIDS would develop common and unusual infections endemic to his or her area of residence. So these clinical differences are not a reason to declare African AIDS different; to say otherwise is an indication of lack of understanding of the disease process. There is nothing unique about the genetic make up of Africans that makes them more susceptible to AIDS (Duh, 1991).

AIDS In Africa: Genetics Versus The Environment

Very early in the HIV/AIDS epidemic, it became clear that black people were disproportionately affected. The much higher prevalence among black Americans, Caribbean blacks, and black Africans, coupled with the notion that clinical presentation of African AIDS patients is different, led to the suggestion that black people are more susceptible to HIV/AIDS. Being more susceptible implies that there is something genetically different about black people that leads to that susceptibility.The question of genetic markers and HIV/AIDS was raised.

A genetic marker that has been associated with susceptibility to disease is one called *Human Leukocyte Antigen* (HLA) complex. An association between HIV/AIDS and HLA has been identified in at least two clinical situations. The HLA-DR5 has been found in patients with Kaposi's sarcoma, and patients who possessed HLA-B35 progressed to AIDS more quickly (Scorza-Smeraldi et al, 1986). But the first association of genetic markers with HIV/ AIDS and black people was that of the marker known as *group specific component* (Gc).

The Gc gene is a glycoprotein found on cells and in serum. It possesses three distinct alleles: Gc 1 fast (Gc 1f), Gc 1 slow (Gc 1s), and Gc 2 distributed in populations by classical Mendelian inheritance; that is, an individual may be heterozygous or homozygous. Homozygous (possessing two copies of the gene) makes one more susceptible to a particular disease (Duh, 1991).

A study by Eales *et al* found a positive association between Gc 1f and AIDS clinical symptoms but a negative association between Gc 2 and AIDS symptoms among homosexuals. The conclusion

117

was that Gc 1f might enhance progression to AIDS, whereas Gc 2 might be protective. They later found higher levels of Gc 1f and lower levels of Gc 2 among American blacks and blacks in Central Africa; the opposite was found among white people. They then speculated that the high frequency of Gc 1f (the susceptibility gene) and low frequency of Gc 2 (the protective gene) in blacks might explain the high prevalence of HIV/AIDS in black populations (Eales *et al*, 1987). A subsequent study by Giles et al (1986) and Daiger *et al* (1987) failed to find an association between Gc and AIDS. Yet the earlier study by Eales *et al* has been quoted as reason for blacks' susceptibility to AIDS (Duh, 1991).

The notion of genetic susceptibility of blacks to HIV/AIDS has been challenged on the basis that the actual research on the correlation between Gc and AIDS was done on homosexual men in Europe. Some Africans have accused the Eales group of implying that there is something genetically wrong with Africans regarding AIDS (Konotey-Ahulu, 1987). In an earlier publication, I maintained that there may or may not be a genetic basis of HIV/AIDS. But environmental factors play a more important role than genetics in the prevalence rates among blacks (Duh, 1991).

In the first place, genetics is not likely because of the distribution of HIV/AIDS in different black populations. For example, in the United States rate among blacks in northeastern states such as New York and New Jersey were higher than in California. In individual states, it was higher in big cities than in rural areas. And within cities, it was higher in the inner city than suburbs. Finally, in every state, the rate was higher among the poor, less educated, less employed members of that race (Duh,

1991). A similar situation existed in Africa. It is higher in the southern part of the continent than the western part. It is higher in metropolitan than rural areas. And there is demonstrated correlation between prevalence and socioeconomic status.

A genetic disease would not have such a distribution. For example, sickle cell disease, a genetic disease that occurs almost exclusively among black people, has a similar prevalence in poor and affluent communities. Furthermore, a gene defect requires the right environmental factors to express itself as a disease, an example being the disease of alcoholism.

Alcoholism is believed to be a genetic disease because of its high prevalence in certain families. Suppose there is gene or chromosomal defect, which then expresses itself as the disease in people who carry that defective gene or chromosome. Those people must have an unrestricted access to alcohol for the disease to manifest itself. Suppose someone is born and lives all his life in a country where alcohol consumption is prohibited by law (as it is in Saudi Arabia). If this individual lives in the country all his life, he would not be exposed to alcohol, and will not develop alcoholism. The genetic defect in this case would be meaningless (Duh, 1991).

The discussion in the last few paragraphs is meant to make two points: (a) there is no clear scientific evidence that black people are genetically susceptible to HIV/AIDS; (b) even if the Gc 1f gene is related to incidence of HIV/AIDS and there is a high frequency of the gene among black people, it does not explain the prevalence rates in Africa. I contend that socioeconomic status is the determining factor. It must be emphasized that socioeconomic status, not just poverty is the key.

119

Does Poverty Cause AIDS?

Does poverty cause AIDS? The answer depends upon how one defines *cause*. If cause is defined in social terms, then the answer is yes. Even with that definition the statement should be poverty *can cause*, not poverty *causes* AIDS. If cause is defined in biological terms as in causative agent, then it is a resounding *no!* But why is there talk in many quarters about poverty being the cause? Does AIDS occur only among poor people? It is truly sad that twenty years into the epidemic and more than 15 years after HIV was discovered as the causative agent, people are still talking about the topic. So-called AIDS dissidents and others have been fueling this notion with potentially harmful consequences. People who have been reluctant to change their risky behavior may decide it is okay to continue those behaviors if they are not going to contract a deadly virus.

It is true that AIDS is devastating sub-Saharan Africa, and Africa has more poor people than any other continent. It is true that in the United States blacks are disproportionately affected by AIDS, and blacks have much higher poverty rates than whites. But it is also true that there is a much higher rate of homosexuality among whites; that white homosexuals tend to be better educated, have better paying jobs, and have higher than average income in the US; that AIDS started in the homosexual community with the potential of wiping out that community but for their aggressive and effective activism.

With the combination of effective educational campaign and antiretroviral therapy, the prevalence of AIDS decreased dramatically in that community. Indeed, white homosexuals are more able to afford the very expensive medications or have insurance that pays for them. But by the end of the year 2000 the prevalence among white homosexuals was going back up. This was partly because of relaxed attitude on the part of young homosexuals regarding preventive measures and the fact that the antiretroviral medications are not as effective due to resistance and other factors. Clearly something other than poverty caused the explosion of AIDS in the homosexual community. And that something is a virus called human immunodeficiency virus—HIV.

The situation with American homosexuals vis-à-vis AIDS weakens the argument that poverty causes AIDS. It is also a strong argument that HIV causes AIDS. As soon as the virus was discovered and means of transmission were identified, they started taking measures to prevent the transmission. Then when the first medications became available, they quickly availed themselves of the medicines to slow the possible decimation of their community. Finally, when HAART became available, they seized the opportunity to stop the decimation of their community. AIDS was no more a major threat to them. Then complacency set in. Because of powerful medications to "cure" the disease, and because of infiltration of the community by AIDS dissidents, some of them abandoned the preventive measures, and the positive trends started being reversed.

What about the situation in Africa? It has become popular in some quarters in Africa and in Europe and America to say that AIDS in Africa is the result of poverty. Yes, it is true that AIDS is devastating Africa and Africa is the poorest continent on earth.

But it is also true that some countries in Africa are poorer than others, and some countries are among the most economically developed and politically stable countries in the developing world. Indeed, many of these countries have urban areas that resemble those in the US and Europe (Halperin, 2000).

As stated earlier, the highest prevalence rates of HIV/AIDS in Africa are in countries in the southern part of the continent. But southern Africa is the most economically developed part of sub-Saharan Africa. Fully 40% of all economic activity in sub-Saharan Africa is generated in the country of South Africa alone. Its per capita income surpasses almost all countries on the continent. And it has one of the highest literacy rates. By the argument that poverty causes AIDS, South Africa should have one of the lowest prevalence rates of HIV/AIDS on the continent. But with 4.7 million sufferers South Africa had the largest number of people living with the condition in the world by the end of 2000. And the disease is spreading there faster than anywhere else on earth. Ironically and sadly, the president of South Africa, Thabo Mbeki, has been at the forefront of those who claim poverty is the cause of AIDS (BBC News, 2000).

Another southern African country in a seemingly paradoxical situation as South Africa is Botswana. Blessed with abundant mineral resources and wildlife, Botswana has the highest per capita income in Africa. It has effective health care and educational systems, both guaranteed to all citizens. It has been very stable politically since independence in 1966 with hardly any corruption. Formal prostitution, a practice by many African women as a means of economic survival, is rare in Botswana. And traditional maladies in tropical Africa such as malnutrition, tuberculosis, and malaria are almost non-existent (Halperin). Yet with 36% of its people living with HIV/AIDS, Botswana had the highest HIV/AIDS prevalence in the world by 2000. Clearly if poverty is the cause of AIDS, then the two richest countries in the region would not have the largest incidence and prevalence rates respectively in the world.

What about the poorest countries? Some countries in West Africa such as Mali, Niger, and Burkina Faso are among the poorest nations on earth, but their prevalence rates were all below 10%. Indeed, Mali, Niger, the Gambia, Guinea, and Senegal, Mauritania, all had rates below 2%. Even Sierra Leone and Liberia, poor countries to begin with, whose economies have been destroyed by protracted civil wars, had rates below 3% (see table 5.2). Furthermore, in Ghana for example, the poorest regions are the three northern regions (Northern, Upper East and Upper West Regions), yet they have the three lowest prevalence rates of the 10 regions of the country. Interestingly, the Cote d'Ivoire was the only country in West Africa with a prevalence of above 10% by December 2000. Yet until recently, Cote d'Ivoire was the most politically stable country and had the most prosperous economy in West Africa. Cote d'Ivoire has persistently led all countries in West Africa in the number of reported cases of AIDS since reporting began in 1986.

So here we are. We hear that poverty is the cause of AIDS, not HIV. Africa is burning because of rampant poverty. By that belief AIDS should occur only among the poor. As discussed above, this theory does not hold water; AIDS is found in rich communities and countries. One can almost say that in some cases wealth is more of a risk for AIDS than poverty, as demonstrated by the prevalence rates in West Africa and Southern Africa.

I stated at the beginning of this section that if one defines cause biologically then it is false to say that poverty causes AIDS. In biological terms, a disease cannot occur when the cause is eliminated. That is, in the case of AIDS people who are not poor cannot get it. Since this is obviously not the case, then the theory that poverty causes AIDS is a weak one, to say the least. Biological basis of cause and effect regarding disease can be explained by an ecological view (Blum, 1976).

An ecological view of a disease involves the consideration of the natural history of the disease. Natural history means the course of the disease—what happens to the individual from the point of contraction to the end of the disease process unaffected by treatment. Without treatment, a disease may end in full recovery, temporary or permanent disability, or death. Which end product of disease is realized depends a lot upon the ecosystem; that is, the individual and his or her environment. This is because the natural history of a disease is a continuum that begins before that individual is exposed to a causative agent to the end of the disease process (see Figure 5.1).

Susceptibility is obviously the most important stage in this continuum. It is the stage before exposure to a causative agent. After exposure, however, susceptibility determines the progression through the continuum. The pre-symptomatic stage occurs when the individual has been exposed to the causative agent. If the agent is an infectious one, it is the stage when infection has taken

124

```
                                              Recovery
                                                ↗
                                               /
Susceptibility  →  Pre-symptomatic  →  Clinical
                   Disease              Disease
                                               \
                                                ↘
                                              Disability or
```

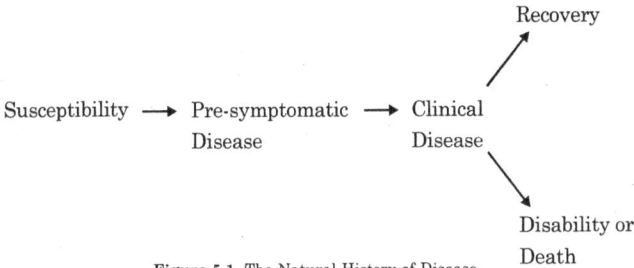

Figure 5.1. The Natural History of Disease Death

place, when the organism has "set up housekeeping" in the host. The organism reproduces itself and thereby causes tissue and/or organ damage. As tissue destruction progresses, the host may have characteristic symptoms and signs of the particular disease the clinical disease stage is reached. The clinical disease stage may end in complete recovery, chronic disability, or death (Duh, 1991).

Susceptibility is determined by individual (host) factors and environmental (biological, physical, and social) factors. It is related to the epidemiological triangle (see Figure 5.2). The triangle being equilateral in shape implies a dynamic relationship among the three components. The dynamic equilibrium may be changed and thereby influence a disease's progression (positively or negatively) if there is significant change in any of the components.

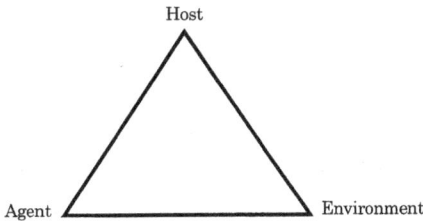

```
                    Host


                     /\
                    /  \
                   /    \
                  /      \
                 /        \
        Agent   /_____\   Environment
```

Figure 5.2. Epidemiological Triangle (Equilateral Triangle)

Changes in the host involve intrinsic factors that may be genetic as well as environmental factors inside the host. Genetic factors have been discussed earlier in the chapter. Environmental factors inside the host may be existing infectious and other diseases, immunological status, and nutritional status. Environmental factors outside the host may be biological (such as plants and animals for food), physical (such as chemical pollutants), and social (such as education, employment, and poverty). The intrinsic factors of the host are influenced by outside environmental factors. When the dynamic equilibrium is disturbed, then the host may become susceptible to the causative agent (Blum, 1974). But the host must be exposed to the agent before infection can occur (the pre-symptomatic disease stage). Whether there is progression to symptomatic disease and death or recovery depends upon the dose and virulence of the agent versus the host factors. (Recall the "dam theory").

The discussion on the ecological view and epidemiological triangle above has hopefully explained the principle of cause and effect. The relationships between intrinsic factors of the host and outside environmental factors have been elucidated. The importance of susceptibility has been stated. But the most important factor in the principle of cause and effect is that the host must be exposed to a causative agent. By that assertion, those who claim that poverty is the cause of AIDS are saying in effect that exposure to poverty leads to the disease AIDS. In other words, the causative agent step in the Natural History diagram is poverty.

I do not believe anyone disputes the fact that poverty contributes to the acquisition of AIDS. What the debate between the "traditionalists" and the "dissidents" is about is the assertion by the dissidents that HIV does not cause AIDS. Those of us in the traditionalist camp are surprised that with all the evidence available, the dissidents maintain that view. As stated by Professor Hoosen Coovadia, the South African chairman of the XIII International AIDS Conference in Durban, South Africa, "to deny that HIV causes AIDS is like saying that the sun rises in the north" (BBC News, 2000).

It should be obvious to those who believe HIV causes AIDS that HIV is the causative agent in the Natural History diagram. And poverty may be the susceptibility factor...*may* because not only poor people are susceptible to the virus. But if poverty is what made a particular individual susceptible to the virus, then poverty will effect the progression from the pre-symptomatic stage to possible death.

There has been a lot of scientific evidence, mostly in monkeys, that clearly indicate that HIV is the cause of AIDS. But the AIDS dissidents maintain that there is no real proof that HIV is the cause of AIDS, that the research in monkeys involving SIV (simian immunodeficiency virus) cannot be translated to humans. The dissidents have included prominent scientists such as Dr. Peter Duesberg of University of California at Berkley and Dr. Charles Thomas of the Helicon Foundation in California, both the United States. Dr. Duesberg has been saying for years that there is no evidence that HIV causes AIDS. He has maintained that drugs is the cause.

These scientists and others have been able to convince many people, including the president of a big country, Thabo Mbeki of South Africa, to join the ranks of the dissidents. In September 2000 Mr. Mbeki stated in parliament that he believed a virus could never cause a syndrome. He would not accept that HIV causes AIDS unless it was proved by a panel of experts he had set up (BBC News, 2000). Significantly, many of the members of the panel were from the dissidents' camp.

It was quite a challenge for the panel to prove that HIV causes AIDS. Scientists in the traditionalist camp maintain that the only absolute way to prove that HIV causes AIDS is to inject the virus into people who do not have AIDS and wait to see if they developed it. This approach is obviously not something scientists are eager to embark on because of the ethical implications. It is even doubtful that there are people who would volunteer to be injected if scientist were willing to carry out such an experiment.

Outside of an ironclad scientific proof, there is a lot of epidemiologic evidence for the HIV-AIDS connection. The simplest evidence is that almost everyone who has had AIDS has tested positive for the HIV since the virus has been isolated. The more convincing evidence is the response to antiretroviral medications. Before the discovery of AZT, most AIDS patients died from opportunistic infections within 1-2 years after diagnosis. When AZT and the other antiretroviral medications became available, they had fewer opportunistic infections and lived longer. Then with the introduction of the PIs, people actually started talking about a cure for the disease. By being on HAART, the patients had virtually no opportunistic infections; they felt stronger and lived longer, and some even went back to work. In the United States, the death rate from AIDS decreased by 47% from 1996 to 1997 because of HAART (Land, 2000).

It is important to note that the use of these drugs is for HIV only; they do not treat the opportunistic infections. Also, those who responded to these medications had lower viral load than those not on medication. Furthermore, those not on HAART had higher viral loads, more opportunistic infections, and died more quickly (van der Horst and Wohl, 2000). But the rate of decline in the deaths in the United States has been slowing as the virus has become resistant to the medications and some patients have stopped taking them because of side effects.

During the XIII International AIDS Conference in Durban, South Africa, in July 2000, several prominent scientists appealed to Mr. Mbeki to change his stance on the issue. The former president of South Africa, Nelson Mandela, also made a similar appeal to Mr. Mbeki but he would not change his mind. He made his declaration that a virus could not cause a syndrome in September. Because of his belief, he would not make available antiretroviral medications to pregnant women in his country when there was clear evidence that they could prevent mother to child transmission.

So the debate went on in Africa and elsewhere between AIDS dissidents and traditionalists. Meanwhile, Africa was burning because of AIDS; and nowhere was the burning more apparent than Mr. Mbeki's South Africa. Finally, his famous panel of experts disbanded in April 2001, having been unable to come up with the proof the president wanted. He seemed to back down on his stance. Indeed, Mr. Mbeki started to "see the light" before his panel concluded its work. He travelled to Cuba in March 2001, where he signed a series of agreements with President Castro to clear the way for Cuba and South Africa to cooperate in producing low-cost generic antiretroviral drugs in the face of the very expensive drugs that were currently available.

REFERENCES

1. BBC News (a). AIDS: Mandela takes on Mbeki. Available at **www.news.bbc.co.uk**. Accessed on 10/21 /2000.
2. BBC News (b). Pressure on Mbeki over AIDS. Available at **www.news.bbc.co.uk**. Accessed on 10/21 /2000.
3. Blum, HL (1974). *Planning for Health: Developmental Application of Social Change*. New York: Human Science Press.
4. Brown, LR (2001). Pandemic produces a missing generation, a population of orphans, shortage of women. *Global AIDS Link*; 65: 6-7.
5. Clumeck, N (1986). Epidemiological correlation between African AIDS and AIDS in Europe. *Infection;* 14: 97-99.
6. Daiger, SP et al (1987). Genetic susceptibility to AIDS: absence of an association with group specific component (Gc). *New England Journal of Medicine*; 317: 631-632.
7. Duh, SV (1991). *Blacks and AIDS: Causes and Origins*; Newbury Park: Sage Publications.
8. Eales LJ, Nye K et al (1987). Group specific component and HIV infection. *Lancet*; 2: 1187-1189.
9. Eales LJ, Parkin JM et al (1987). Association of different allelic forms of group specific component with susceptibility to and clinical manifestation of humanimmuno deficiency virus infection. *Lancet*; 1: 999-1002.
10. Enlow, RW et al (1983). Increased frequency of HLA-DR5 in lymphadenopathy stage of AIDS. *Lancet*; 1: 51.

11. Giles, K et al (1987). Genetic susceptibility to AIDS: absence of an association with group specific component (Gc). *New England Journal of Medicine*; 317: 630-631.

12. Halperin, D (2001). Is poverty the root cause of African AIDS? *AIDSLink*; 65, 9.

13. Konotey-Ahulu, FID (1987a). Group-specific component and HIV infection. *Lancet*; 1: 1287.

14. Konotey-Ahulu, FID (1987b). AIDS in Africa: misinformation and disinformation. *Lancet*; 2: 206-207.

15. Lands, L. Beyond eradication. *POZ*; 3/2000: 62-63

16. Last, JM (Ed) (1983). *A Dictionary of Epidemiology*; New York: Oxford University Press.

17. Scorza-Smeraldi, RS (1986). HLA-associated susceptibility to acquired immunodeficiency syndrome in Italian patients with human immunodeficiency virus. *Lancet*; 2: 1187-1189.

18. UNAIDS (2001a). HIV/AIDS in Africa. Available at **www.unaids.org**. Accessed on 2/2/2001.

19. UNAIDS (2001b). The interplay of factors driving sexual transmission. Available at **www.unaids.org.** Accessed on 29 /1/01.

20. UNAIDS (2005). AIDS epidemic update: sub-Saharan Africa. Available at **www.unaids.org.** Accessed on 10/5/06

20. van der Horst C, Wohl DA. Opportunistic infections in the era of HAART.*Conference Summaries from the XIII International AIDS Conference. July 9-14, 2000, Durban, South Africa*; 31-40.

CHAPTER SIX

AFRICA IS BURNING

From July 9 to14, 2000, an unprecedented event took place on the continent of Africa. For six memorable days, over 13,000 scientists, politicians, AIDS activists, people living HIV/AIDS and other delegates gathered in Durban, South Africa for the XIII International AIDS Conference. The significant thing about this event is that it was the first of these conferences to be held in the developing world. But more importantly, it took place in the epicentre of the HIV/AIDS pandemic. With more than 70% of the HIV/AIDS cases in the world, Africa definitely deserved the attention such a conference brought, and South Africa deserved to be the host country, being the country with the largest number of HIV/AIDS sufferers in the world.

The theme of the conference was "Break the Silence". The theme was appropriate because Africa was slowly being consumed by HIV/AIDS while the rest of the world remained silent, while multinational drug companies remained silent about the unavailability of HIV medications in Africa, while many governments on the continent remained silent about the devastation of the epidemic in their countries. The theme was also meant to break the silence about the stigma surrounding HIV/AIDS and the denial by some that HIV causes AIDS. But an unofficial theme of the conference was "Africa is Burning" as many AIDS activists wore T-shirts bearing that inscription.

The slogan "Africa is burning" was first unveiled as AIDS activists shouted it over and over at the conclusion of the XII International AIDS Conference in Geneva, Switzerland, in 1998. The slogan was mainly directed at the multinational drug companies for not making life-saving medications available and affordable to African HIV/AIDS sufferers. So why is Africa burning? Is it because there are no drugs to treat HIV/AIDS? Before tackling this question, the question of whether Africa is burning needs to be addressed first.

Africa, the poorest continent on earth, has been "burning" slowly, maybe "simmering", for a long time. Its 53 independent countries and over 600 million population have been marginalized for generations. Many of these countries had to fight wars against colonial masters for their independence. In some of these countries such as the Congo, South Africa, and Zimbabwe, different African factions fought each other in addition to fighting the colonialists. Then after independence, civil wars within countries and territorial wars between countries sprang up in almost every part of the continent. In countries like Angola, Sudan, and Liberia these wars went on for more than a decade.

Beside wars, political instability has been the order of the day in Africa. Corruption, unequal distribution of wealth, and tribalism have led to numerous *coups d'etat* across the continent. Economic mismanagement and inefficiency along with unfair trade practices by economic superpowers have robbed Africa of a lot of her natural resources. Then, there have been frequent episodes of drought causing massive famines in some countries. With their economies in shambles, most of these countries borrowed heavily from developed countries and international financial institutions like the World Bank and International Monetary Fund (1MF). And many of these countries have been spending up to 50% of their GDP on servicing foreign debts.

With so much being spent on debt repayment, coupled with wars, droughts, mismanagement and corruption, there was little resource available for development projects including health care infrastructure. In real terms, government health budgets shrunk by about 50% by the 1980s (Tawfit, 2000). In addition to material resources, Africa has been losing human resources through the "brain drain" phenomenon. Intellectually and technically trained young people, many of them trained at government expense, have been leaving in their numbers for greener pastures overseas. So from independence in the 1960s to the early 1980s, Africa had been simmering, burning slowly.

Africa had been burning slowly from huge foreign debts, droughts, the brain drain phenomenon, and economic and political instability. Africa had been burning slowly from poverty, malnutrition, and infectious diseases. Tuberculosis, malaria, and diarrhoeal diseases had been killing millions of Africans. Then a new disease called Acquired Immunodeficiency Syndrome, AIDS, sprang itself onto the continent in the form of an epidemic. The fire that had been simmering, burning slowly as underbrush, became fuelled by the AIDS epidemic. Through denial, complacency, and lack of resources (human and material), the underbrush has become a full-blown forest fire. Meanwhile, some countries had achieved some degree of economic progress and political stability prior to the arrival of AIDS on the scene.

The tragedy about the HIV/AIDS epidemic in Africa is its potential to wipe out the modest and even substantial progress made by some countries. It also has the potential to decimate whole populations in some parts of the continent. It has the potential to produce more political and economic instability, disturb social structure, and transform the cultural landscape of the continent. In several countries, particularly those in the southern part of the continent, the potential for disaster is very real indeed. Yes; Africa is burning because of HIV/AIDS. But I contend that it is not because of unavailability of expensive antiretroviral medications.

As stated in the last chapter, the AIDS epidemic in Africa was manageable by 1990. By that year, fewer than three million Africans might have been living with HIV/AIDS; ten years later, the number was a whopping 25.3 million. And Africa had buried 17 million of the 21.8 million people worldwide who had died of AIDS since the epidemic began. How did this happen? What factors contributed to this massive explosion? As in other parts of the world, many factors contributed to the spread of HIV/AIDS, but the transmission process is a major factor in the explosion of cases in Africa. As discussed in earlier chapters of the book, sexual (heterosexual) activity is the main mode of HIV transmission in Africa, and the explosion is not due to genetic factors. Two main factors influence the sexual transmission—biological and socio-economic.

It has to be understood that for a disease to spread, the causative agent has to be present in the population and the right conditions have to be present for the causative agent to propagate itself. In the case HIV/AIDS the virus (causative agent) has firmly established itself on the continent of Africa, certainly in sub-Saharan Africa. And the right conditions for the virus to propagate itself and spread exist in the form of biological and socio-economic factors.

Biological Factors

To understand how the biological factors affect the HIV/AIDS epidemic, we need to review the process of HIV transmission and the pathogenesis of AIDS. It was discussed in Chapter Three that the transmission and pathogenesis depend upon a person's state of health before exposure to HIV. The virus needs an effective portal of entry in order to get into the body and establish housekeeping; that is, to establish an infection. Once the infection is established, the person's general health status determines how fast HIV infection progresses to AIDS, and the most important aspect of the health status is the quality of the immune system. Recall that the skin and mucous membranes provide the first line of defence, and the immune system takes over once the organism has entered the body.

HIV Transmission.

When it comes to heterosexual transmission of HIV, sexually transmitted infections (STIs) provide effective portals of entry. Diseases such as syphilis, Chancroid, and herpes cause genital ulcers through which the virus could pass into the body. Other STIs such as gonorrhoea and chlamydia produce inflammation that compromises the integrity of vaginal and urethral mucosae and creates a portal of entry into the body (Duh, 1991). Another risk for effective portal of entry is the uncircumcised penis. The foreskin is vulnerable to STIs because it is more difficult to keep clean. Also, HIV spreads more easily by means of immune receptors called *Langerhans cells* that are highly concentrated in the foreskin of the uncircumcised penis (Halperin, 2000).

There is a very high prevalence of STIs in many African countries. Furthermore, many of these STIs go untreated or are inadequately treated because of inefficient health care systems. In addition, some genital ulcers like syphilis and herpes may not hurt or may go away without treatment. Because they do not hurt or may go away on their own, people with these genital ulcers may not seek treatment. In the meantime, they may be involved in multiple sexual partnerships, increasing their chance of acquiring HIV or transmitting it to others. On the other hand, there is a low rate of male circumcision in many African countries, particularly countries in southern parts of the continent (UNAIDS, 2001). So it appears that high prevalence of STIs in males and females, and low rates of male circumcision are two major factors for sexual transmission of HIV in Africa.

Pathogenesis of AIDS.

Once HIV enters the body, it goes on a relentless pursuit of propagating itself by destroying the body's immune system. It uses the CD4 cells to reproduce itself, and when the CD4 count falls to below 200 cells/ml, the person becomes vulnerable to various opportunistic infections. Obviously, how soon one goes from HIV infection to below 200 CD4 count depends upon how many CD4 cells there are to begin with.

The CD4 count, indeed the whole immune system, is related to the general health status of the individual, nutritional status, environmental stresses, and existence of other diseases, particularly certain infectious diseases. With regard to the last factor, research has shown that some infectious diseases tend to stimulate the immune system, and stimulated CD4 cells are easier targets for HIV destruction. Infections such as syphilis, cytomegalovirus (CMV), Epstein-Barr virus (EBV), and herpes simplex virus stimulate the immune system. And research has shown that in populations with high rates of these and other infections, there is also a high prevalence of HIV/AIDS (Duh, 1991).

The four risk factors listed above are rather common in Africa. That is, there is a high rate of general poor health, poor nutritional status, a lot of environmental stress, and many infectious diseases that are endemic. Diseases such as malaria, tuberculosis, and gastroenteritis place a lot of stress on the immune system. Because these and other endemic diseases are so common in most of Africa, the immune system of most Africans is weakened by constantly battling endemic diseases. Therefore, HIV has an easier time infecting and destroying their CD4 cells.

Another biological factor of the pathogenic process is the viral load. The number of HIV in the blood stream tends to be highest at the beginning stages of infection. Then the viruses enter tissue where they may lie dormant or destroy CD4 cells. It is again very high at the late stages of illness when the viruses have had a chance to multiply over and over. The danger about this phenomenon is that an infected person is more likely to infect others at the early stages of HIV infection because of high viral load. And this is the time the infected person may not know that he or she is infected.

Socio-economic Factors

The biological factors discussed above are influenced and perpetuated by socio-economic factors, the most prominent of which is multiple sexual partnerships. Multiple sexual activities, of course, leads to the spread of STIs that can lead to the consequences of HIV/AIDS as discussed above. And multiple sexual partnerships are very common in many African countries.

The idea of multiple sexual partnerships is related to polygamy—more specifically polygeny. *Polygeny* is the cultural practice that permits men to have as many wives as they want but does not allow women to have more than one husband. From ancient times, African men have had the privilege of having more than one wife. In the olden days, having more than one wife was not necessarily a sexual matter but an economic one.

In the olden days when agriculture was the main or only economic activity in most African countries, manual labour was the only means available to cultivate the crops or raise livestock. Obviously, the more people there were to work on the farm, the more land could be cultivated and the higher the yield of the crops. Since by tradition land ownership was the domain of men, they controlled the labour force. Therefore, a man married several women to have many children to work on the farm. Often wealthier men had several farms and needed more people to work on the farms, so they tended to have more wives and children than average. Indeed, a man's wealth was viewed in terms of the number of wives and children he had, in addition to his material possessions. Such a man commanded a lot of respect in his town or village. Such a man would labelled a "big man" (Duh, 1999).

The practice of polygeny had a spillover effect. As time went on, a practice that started as an economic matter evolved to become a sexual matter. In fact, it became a matter of exercising power and control over women. Therefore, it was not uncommon for a man with several wives to have extramarital relationships. Women and girls who responded to such men were often rewarded with monetary and other gifts. Since men controlled most of the available property, women were often economically marginalized. For their economic survival, therefore, unmarried women often yielded to the sexual advances of wealthy married men.

During the late colonial and early post-independence era, economic activity became more diversified. Exporting of raw materials such as cocoa, coffee, and timber, and the mining of Africa's abundant mineral reserves required a workforce outside of farming. Formal education became a necessity to produce the requisite workforce. And formal education further diversified the economy as teachers, lawyers, doctors, clerical staff, and other technicians were produced.

The diversification of the economy led to fewer family-run activities like farming. Therefore, a man did not need so many wives and children to help him. Besides, children wanted to go to school, and some governments in the newly independent countries made education compulsory for all school-age children. So it became a burden for a man to have many children. The practice of polygeny became less and less. By the early 1980s when AIDS reared its ugly head, fewer than 20% of men in most African countries had more than one wife (Duh, 1999). However, multiple sexual partnerships did not fade away with the practice of polygeny.

When men realized that they could not or should not have several wives, they satisfied their sexual desire by having overlapping relationships. So a man with one wife might have a girl friend or two on the side. An unmarried man might have one girl friend and a casual partner or two on the side. Again, women and girls responded to men mostly for economic reasons. Also because of lack of social power, some women and girls felt obliged to respond to men irrespective of economic need. Obviously, the foregoing does not mean that there was no love involved in sexual relationships.

In addition to the situations discussed above, sexuality per se has been socially sanctioned in African society as it has been in other societies. Being sexually active is a ritualistic passing from teenager to adulthood. In many African countries, teenagers and young adults are encouraged to be sexually active. The practice started in the olden days when people got married in their late teens or early 2Os. Even girls' getting married in their early teens was not uncommon. But because of education few people in the post-independence era get married at such a young age. Still they are encouraged to be sexually active.

There are also some beliefs and myths which perpetuate this phenomenon. There is a self-imposed and peer pressure to be sexually active at a young age. That is, some young people might believe that others might think they are abnormal if they are a virgin; and some may actually be told by peers that there is something wrong with them if they do not have sex. Again, self-imposed and peer pressure to be sexually active is not unique to Africans; it is quite a universal phenomenon. But sexual myths may be more common in African societies.

In my travels in Ghana in the late 1990s, I had a chance to talk with young people about the pressures many of them felt to engage in sex. Male teenagers might be told by their friends that sexual activity would make the penis larger, and women and girls prefer a bigger penis. In this regard, the earlier virginity is broken and the more frequently one engaged in sex, the larger the penis would become. Furthermore, a big penis would become small and a small penis would become even smaller if one did not have sex. On secondary school and university campuses, male virgins would be teased and labelled as queer. Some virgins would lie about their virginity so as to avoid being teased. At the University of Ghana, students were labelled "munchers" and "chewers"…munchers being those with at least one active sexual partner, and chewers being those without. It means that there was a misguided view that munchers were "somebody" and chewers were suffering because they could not even manage to acquire a sexual partner on campus. Clearly, there was some kind of pressure on the chewers to become munchers, and for the munchers, the higher the number of partners the better.

Another myth among Ghanaian men is that having sex with younger women or girls makes for a freer bowel movement. In other words, this is a way to prevent or treat constipation. So older men like to have sex with teenage girls. One man in his 40s said to me with pride, pointing at a young woman in a small town: "I was the first man to have her . . . she was a virgin then. I got her pregnant, and since then no other man has been able to get her pregnant". A recent myth in some parts of Africa is that a man with HIV infection could rid himself of the virus by having sex with a virgin. Such men would give money to school girls and have sex with them without revealing their HIV status. This phenomenon has accelerated the rate of raping young girls in countries like Kenya and South Africa. This is a very dangerous myth indeed.

Female virgins also suffer from teasing and being called queer on campuses. They are pressured to have sex out of a sense of duty, respect, or fear often with older men. One university student in Ghana told me that she was pressured by fellow students to break her virginity before she was ready. While she was in secondary school, she was told by several female friends that she would become ill or mentally retarded if she did not have sex. Others told her that her vaginal canal would be closed up without sex, and she would not be able to have children if she waited too long. One friend told her of the many benefits of an active sex life, including the fact that sex made a girl put on weight. (Being relatively heavy is a sign of beauty in many African societies). This student had planned to remain a virgin until she got married, but she was convinced by friends that it was dangerous to her health to wait that long.

Various beliefs and myths pertaining to sexuality had existed in African societies, as they had in other societies, when the AIDS epidemic started. Because of the existence of the biological factors discussed earlier, the epidemic took hold and spread quite quickly. The biological factors were in turn influenced by socio-economic factors. For example, malnutrition and poor general health are related to poverty; and the very high prevalence of STIs has to do in part with the culture of multiple sexual partnerships. Having discussed some possible reasons behind multiple sexual partnerships in Africa, we need to discuss some of the other socio-economic factors that perpetuate the phenomenon.

Another legacy of the colonial era regarding the diversification of the economy is the spread of STIs. The introduction of education and industries required that people leave their hometowns for distant places to work in the new industries or attend boarding schools. Men left their wives and girlfriends at home to work in mines and other industries to sustain the growing urbanization. They were gone for lengthy periods of time; and the long absences from their wives and girlfriends attracted them to prostitutes. The same urbanization process attracted women to the growing cities. With fewer job opportunities for them, many of the women indulged in formal and informal prostitution. The multiple sexual partnership involved in prostitution fermented the spread of STIs. Then these urban dwellers travelled back and forth to their hometowns and spread STIs there (Dawson, 1988; Duh, 1991). A similar situation existed for young people who attended boarding school far from their hometown.

The idea of leaving the hometown for lengthy periods persisted in the post-independence era. Industries such as mining required workers to be away from their partners for long periods of time. Meanwhile, industrialization required effective rail and road transportation. And railway stations and truck stops became centres of prostitution, further promoting the spread of STIs. Indeed, the Trans Africa Highway connecting Kenya, Uganda, Rwanda, Burundi, and the Congo had been largely responsible for the high prevalence of STIs in those countries. It is also believed to be mainly responsible for the high prevalence of HIV/AIDS in East and Central Africa during the early part of the epidemic (Hag, 1988). In addition to work and schooling that led to the migration from one's hometown, prostitution has been supported by tourism, a post independence industry (Duh, 1991). Young women often hang around hotels and other resort areas as full time prostitutes or casual ones, some of them students, to be picked up by tourists who tend to have foreign currency for the women. Port cities where ships dock are particularly noted for this phenomenon.

So when HIV/AIDS was introduced into Africa in the early 1980s, the right conditions, some having origins in the colonial period, were present for its rather fast spread. As stated before, denial, complacency, and lack of resources have permitted those behaviours and conditions to go on in the era of HIV/AIDS. Some of the sexual practices described above are not unique to Africa. For example, pressure from peers to engage in sex is quite common in the developed world. And multiple sexual partnership was the norm during the so-called sexual revolution and drug culture of the 1960s and 70s in the United States and Europe. But the fast spread of the epidemic in Africa has been attributed to the 3 Ps (Polygamy, Prostitution, Poverty) and traditional practices. All these parameters affect women disproportionately; that is, there is a strong gender inequality vis-à-vis the HIV/AIDS epidemic.

As stated in the last chapter, 55% of people living HIV/AIDS in Africa by the end of 2000 were female. In some of the most heavily affected countries, the rate of new infections among young people in the age range 15-19 was five times higher in females than males. Among those in their early 20s, it was three times higher in females. This unfortunate, some say unfair, state of affairs is related to the four parameters listed above. Polygeny as discussed earlier obviously favours males. Thus, women are victims of the system since in many cases, they have little say in sexual matters. Prostitution concerning women is obvious, and more women are affected by poverty (I prefer "socio-economic status"). Finally, traditional practices have always placed African women in subservient roles, as in other societies.

Polygamy

The word *polygamy* means that a man can have as many wives as he wants and a woman can have as many husbands as she wants at the same time. There is no legal or cultural basis for polygamy in Africa. But if one stretches the definition of the word to include all sexual activity between men and women, then polygamy does exist in Africa... as it does in other societies. As stated earlier, the legally sanctioned practice of polygeny is dying out, but men's desire and authority to have several sexual partners has perpetuated the practice. In as much as men can have several women concurrently, and since there are not that many women around to satisfy men's desires, many women necessarily do have more than one male partner; hence the existence of polygamy in a *de facto* manner. Women may practise polygamy formally as prostitutes or informally with casual sexual partners. In both cases, economic dependence on men is often the determining factor. For example, studies conducted in Namibia and South Africa found that women were aware of AIDS but felt unable to stay in a monogamous relationship because of money (Susser and Stein, 2000).

How does economic dependence on men influence women's sexual behaviour? As stated above, I prefer *socio-economic status* to *poverty*. Sociologists define poverty as the chronic inability to provide for basic necessities of life such as food, clothing, and shelter. The United Nations defines it in a similar way in devising poverty reduction programs in developing countries. If one uses the above definition to describe poverty, then many women in urban areas of Africa would not consider themselves poor because they are often able to provide for the basic necessities of life. This is why it is dangerous to say that poverty is what drives women to put themselves at risk. Those who do not consider themselves poor might falsely believe that they are not at risk for HIV/AIDS. Furthermore, with that definition those who claim that poverty is the cause of AIDS would have to think twice if they take a look at the situation in Botswana.

Botswana had the highest per capita income in Africa, yet it had the highest prevalence of HIV/AIDS in the world by end of 2000. Also, South Africa had the largest number of people living with HIV/AIDS in the world, with an estimated 4.7 million cases by the end of 2000; yet it was the richest country in Africa, controlling fully 40% of all economic activity on the continent. And the Cote d'Ivoire was the only country in West Africa with prevalence of over 10% yet it was the most economically stable country in West Africa until recently. So I will illustrate how socio-economic status (not poverty) may cause a woman to indulge in risky behaviour.

Let us look at two prototype women in a relatively politically and economically stable country like Ghana. The first one is a 20-year old university student who left her hometown to live on campus. She has a boyfriend at home, and then she takes one of her classmates as a steady boyfriend on campus. This woman's parents are quite well off and give her enough money for her tuition, room and board, books and incidentals. She is above average in terms of beauty, and she wants to look even more attractive. She keeps two sets of clothing—a few traditional attires and several western ones including dresses, skirts, pairs of trousers, and assorted pairs of imported shoes. She has quite an elaborate make-up kit; and she goes to the beauty salon every couple of weeks to fix her hair. Finally, she likes going to clubs and restaurants off campus. To sustain such a lifestyle, she needs more money than her parents provide, and the boyfriend on campus is unable to offer any financial help. So she gets a "sugar daddy" off campus. When she goes back to her hometown during vacation, she may have a liaison with her old boy friend who may be married.

The second woman is a 25 years old unmarried university graduate. She works for an international airline at the airport in the capital city. Her salary is well above the average of her contemporaries who work for the government. She lives in a nicely decorated rented apartment. She has an even more elaborate set of clothing and make-up kit, and she goes to the beauty salon about once a week. She goes to clubs and restaurants quite often. She has a steady boyfriend who does not make as much money as she. At the end of the month, she does not have enough money to pay her rent and utilities, so she turns to a sugar daddy. When she visits her hometown, she might have a liaison with her old boyfriend who is now married.

In both situations described above, sugar daddy is married, older with a car, and may have another partner besides his wife and this one. Also, old boyfriend at home may have another partner in addition to his wife. And steady boyfriend may not be totally faithful to her. Thus, each of these women may be exposed to more than three sources of infection; they are at a very high risk of contracting HIV and other STIs. However, neither woman is likely to consider herself at risk for HIV infection. After all they have only one steady boyfriend, and they are "clean" well-educated women.

Obviously, neither woman would consider herself poor. She is able to provide for basic necessities. It is her desire for more

149

that drives her to indulge in the risky behaviour. And the scenarios described above are not uncommon in urban areas of Africa. So to say that only poor people get AIDS is a dangerous statement indeed. In fact, I would suggest that it is because of their relative affluence that these fictitious women have that many partners. Had they been relatively poor, they might have been content with a simpler lifestyle and stayed with one partner or none. Similarly, if sugar daddy did not drive a car and have a lot of money to spend on several women, he might have been faithful to his wife. Again, sugar daddy does not consider himself at risk.

One university student in Ghana told me that most of the students, particularly the female students, want to have everything nice for modern living. Some of them take holiday trips to Europe and America and come back with all kinds of lifestyle changes which others try to copy. Many of the female students who live on the university campus want to have everything nice such as mobile phones, refrigerators, colour television, and video cassette player. The desire for those items is even stronger once their leave school. Some of them would get them, in addition to those listed earlier, whether they themselves can afford them or not. And in many cases the only way out for them is to have a sugar daddy. Some of them also frequent the first class hotels to meet foreign tourists who give them money in foreign currencies. So these university students who are not poor and are perceived as "clean" are putting themselves at risk for HIV and others STIs.

Some men falsely believe that so-called clean women do not harbour any infections. Likewise, some women consider married men as "clean"; a single man is more likely to run around. In this regard, men are less likely to use protection during encounters with "clean" women. A study reported in the Population Council's *Studies in Family Planning* of September 2000 found that Nigerian men used condoms more often with prostitutes than with casual sexual partners or their wives.

Perhaps nowhere is wealth a potential risk for HIV infection in Africa than in the country of Botswana. Because of relative affluence, Halperin states that until recently, young people in Botswana were more likely to be killed by a BMW car than by childhood illnesses. Young people have had enough disposable income to frequent nightclubs and live the "good life", and this phenomenon has been continued in the era of HIV/AIDS. However, men tend to control the wealth and women tend to be economically dependent on them. Halperin quotes a man in a focus group in Botswana as saying, "If a girl accepts a beer or two, she is `yours' for the evening. These girls are easy to find. . . and most of them don't worry about condoms, especially after a few drinks." (Halperin, 2000; p. 9). Again I submit that relative wealth, the ability to go to nightclubs, is what puts both Botswanan men and women at risk for HIV infection.

Poverty.

To be sure, there is a definite relationship between poverty and HIV/AIDS. My contention is that it is not the only cause, and poverty per se does not lead to the acquisition of HIV/AIDS. What is clear is that poverty can and does contribute to both the acquisition of HIV and quick progression to AIDS. Poor women are more likely to indulge in prostitution as a means of economic survival. And both men and women are often likely to have risky behaviour if they are poor. Another study reported in the September 2000 *Studies in Family Planning* stated that slum residents in Nairobi (Kenya) initiated sex at an earlier age and had more sexual partners than did other city residents. Obviously then prostitutes and slum dwellers are at a high risk of acquiring and spreading HIV.

Poor people everywhere tend to have poor nutrition, poor hygiene, and poor general health. They tend to get ill more often with the usual endemic diseases; and they are less likely to utilize health care, especially in places where health care institutions are few. So if they are likely to start sex at an earlier age and have multiple partners, then poor people are more likely to have STIs. And STIs provide easy access into the body by HIV. Once infected with HIV, a person with poor general health, poor nutrition, and the existence of other diseases progresses more quickly to AIDS. Thus, such a person has a weakened immune system to begin with and is likely to die from AIDS rather quickly.

Prostitution.

Some of the background information regarding the genesis and perpetuation of prostitution in many African countries has been discussed in this chapter. They mostly parallel the process of urbanization and industrialization in Africa. Like other customs and practices, once prostitution took hold it spread and persisted beyond the initial boundaries and purposes. Thus, in many countries modern day prostitution is not limited to urban areas. Prostitution can be found in most areas, rural and urban, of most countries. And it is mostly driven by women's need of or desire for money.

There are "amateur" prostitutes. In this regard, there are some women who travel to urban and other areas such as mining centres and port areas for short periods of time to engage in prostitution. Such women may need money for specific projects and decide to indulge in this trade for as long as they could accumulate the needed funds, and then they return to their hometown to continue their usual activities. These types of prostitutes may be missed by policies and programs that target prostitutes. And the women themselves may not consider themselves as prostitutes; neither might they consider themselves at risk for HIV infection. Also, the fictitious women discussed earlier, who take sugar daddies for economic reasons, might be considered "amateur prostitutes" if one defines prostitution as exchange of sex for money. I have referred to this phenomenon by the term *transactional sex*. It is instructive to note that the phenomena discussed in this section are not limited to Africa. Transactional sex is a worldwide phenomenon and has contributed a lot toward the spread of HIV/AIDS everywhere.

Traditional practices.

With regard to traditional practices, the practice of polygeny, which has become a de facto polygamy, is perhaps the most significant. Since males usually control sexuality, they often decide when to have sex and with how many females concurrently. Thus one HIV-infected male could infect several females, and if some of them become pregnant, the offspring could be infected also. In other words, a male's risk for HIV infection depends upon the number of sexual partners and frequency of sexual activity, whereas females' risk is largely the result of their male partners' sexual behaviour (Ardayfio, 2000). There are some other traditional practices that are female-centred.

African women are very particular about feminine hygiene. They meticulously wash the vagina with water or water and soap at every bath; and in many cases, they take a bath at least twice a day. They almost ritualistically take a bath before sexual encounter. In some parts of East Africa, some women use locally made herbal medicines to douche (Green et al, 2000). This practice is also common in Ghana. The meticulous cleaning and the douching with herbal medicines have a tendency to dry the vagina, and dry vaginal mucosa tears more easily during intercourse, providing easy access for HIV to enter the blood stream. In addition, soap and other chemicals for douching change the pH of the vagina from a very acidic environment to a more basic one. The natural acidic environment is protective against certain organisms. Therefore, when this is disturbed, the women are at an increased risk for other STIs.

A traditional practice that is common in Zimbabwe and some other African countries is "dry sex". This is when women insert herbs, powders, or other substances to tighten and dry the vagina before intercourse. This is supposed to produce more friction and enhance the men's sensation. Obviously dry sex is a risk for HIV transmission as explained above. Dry sex has been introduced to some other countries in Southern Africa including Botswana, and this practice is believed to be partly responsible for the very high HIV/AIDS prevalence in Botswana (Halperin, 2001).

Another traditional practice that places women at increased risk for HIV infection and other STIs is female circumcision. It is an ancient ritual that has been practised in many countries in the Middle East and Africa through the 20th century. Those who defend the practice say it is equivalent to male circumcision, but women's advocates say that it is far more drastic and damaging than male circumcision. Thus, in the past several years, the practice has been referred to as *Female Genital Mutilation* (FGM).

The term FGM covers three main forms of genital mutilation: (1) *Sunna circumcision* is the removal of the prepuce and/or the tip of the clitoris. (2) *Clitoridectomy* is the removal of the entire clitoris and the adjacent labia. (3) *Infibulation*, the most extreme form, consists of the removal of the clitoris and the adjacent labia, and joining of the scraped sides of the vulva across the vagina. A small opening is left for urination and the flow of menstrual blood; and the woman is cut open to allow intercourse on the night of wedding or other form of marriage (Daileader, 2001)

The practice is often done under unsanitary conditions with unclean sharp instruments such as razor blades, scissors, kitchen knives, and pieces of glass. These instruments are often used on several girls in succession with little cleaning between uses. Antiseptic and other sterilization techniques are not employed. Therefore, this practice often results in infections of the genital and surrounding areas. And the use of unclean instruments on several girls at a time can cause the transmission of HIV and other STIs (Daileader, 2001). Furthermore, the fact that the normal architecture of the vaginal area has been altered could cause easier access to blood by HIV during intercourse with an HIV-infected man.

155

Why is such a risky and painful custom practised? In countries where this is done, it is considered a necessity to usher girls into womanhood. In some parts of Kenya FGM forms part of an elaborate ceremony welcoming the girl into womanhood. It is governed by certain cultural beliefs. For example, an uncircumcised girl is considered "unclean" and cannot be married. A girl whose clitoris is not removed is considered a great danger because if a man's penis touches the clitoris during intercourse, the man would die (Daileader, 2001).

Mostly as a result of pressure from women's advocates outside of Africa, many countries have initiated laws to modify or outlaw FGM. But it goes on in other countries. Remarkably, some of the staunchest supporters of the practice are females. They are unwilling to give up this custom since they have always done it this way. They consider the practice as family honour, cleanliness, and protection against spells; and they do not want it changed (Daileader, 2001).

The male control of sexual matters has another effect, what I call "the nice girl syndrome" That is, there are certain things nice girls are not supposed to do. For example, nice girls are not supposed to have multiple partners, so they would not talk about it if they do. Some even believe that nice girls are not supposed to have premarital sex and would not admit to it. Nice girls are not supposed to approach men romantically, and they are not supposed to initiate discussion on contraceptives. One of the university students in Ghana told me that most girls in secondary school did not discuss contraception with their boyfriends. They were even shy to discuss them with girl friends. For example, a girl might approach another and say something like "A friend of mine at home wants to know what kind of pill to take to prevent pregnancy" or "A friend of mine at home is pregnant. . . do you know where she can get an abortion?" In both situations, the questioner might be talking about herself but would not want to appear as if she is a bad girl.

The nice girl syndrome is really a paradox. Premarital sex is socially sanctioned and approved of in many African societies. Sometimes parents even encourage their children, particularly boys, to have sex. Yet nice girls are not supposed to have sex. It is almost laughable that girls are not supposed to have sex. One has to ask, if boys are encouraged to have sex, with whom are they supposed to do it? Another aspect of the nice girl syndrome is that because of the fact that young people are supposed to respect their elders, girls and young women may not be able to say no to sexual advances by older men. To say no would imply lack of respect for or disobedience to an elder.

Because of the nice girl syndrome, girls often sneak around for sex, particularly when the partner is an older man. As such, they are often not relaxed during intercourse. When a female is not relaxed during intercourse, the vagina tends to be tight, a situation that can lead to mucosal breaks and tears, giving access to HIV transmission. Also, when the female is not relaxed, the natural hormones that are released to lubricate the vagina for intercourse are not properly released; and the dry vagina breaks and tears more easily for easy access to HIV transmission.

Another unfortunate aspect of the nice girl syndrome is illegal abortions. Again, because nice girls are not supposed to have sex, not supposed to get pregnant outside of marriage, they would not tell their parents when pregnancy occurs. They are reluctant to go to the hospital for a medically supervised abortion, lest their parents be told about it. So they may go to a back alley clinic or even someone's house where untrained people perform the abortion under very un-sterile conditions. This often leads to the contraction of all kinds of infections and even death. These kinds of back alley abortions often disturb the normal architecture of the vagina, leading to the risk of HIV and other STI transmission.

Finally, because of the nice girl syndrome, females are reluctant to buy and carry condoms. If they muster the courage to ask the partner to use condom and he refuses, they often give in. Men are also often reluctant to use condoms when they are with "nice girls" because of the belief that those "clean" partners do not carry any infections. Furthermore, some men believe that if they use condoms, the partner might think they are being unfaithful. And there are those men who refuse to use the condom because it reduces sexual pleasure. This last statement is not entirely an African phenomenon; many men in other societies hold the same view.

Men who refuse to use condoms may take a fatalistic attitude and rationalize their behaviour. For example, in a television interview by the Christian Broadcasting Network (CBN) in December 2000, a young man in Zimbabwe stated that he did not like using condoms, and it was okay if he contracted STIs including HIV. He added: "You can die from a car accident; why not AIDS?" A statement by another young man was even more serious...and sad. This was a young man with HIV infection who stated: "I didn't fool around... didn't go looking for it. So I will spread it around".

Another sad and potentially dangerous attitude expressed in the CBN report is the assertion that HIV/AIDS has nothing to do with sex. Evidently many young people in Zimbabwe and other African countries embrace the notion that HIV does not cause AIDS. If HIV does not cause AIDS, then sexual transmission of the virus is a moot point. They claim that AIDS stands for **A**merica's **I**dea to **D**iscourage **S**ex. Some men in Ghana have expressed a similar sentiment. In a focus group discussion by the Forum for African Women Educationalists (FAWE) on knowledge and attitudes about HIV/AIDS, some men in Ghana stated their belief that AIDS is just a scare tactic being used by the Western world to stop people from being promiscuous; and that condom is one of the many tools the white man has produced to manipulate Africans (Armah, 2001). Obviously, people with those kinds of attitudes are not likely to hesitate about multiple sexual partnerships without condoms.

The final traditional practice worth mentioning here is widowhood rites. In many African societies, when a married man dies, his brother or nephew may inherit his property. And his "property" includes his wife or wives. When the inheritor is already married, it means he adds the dead relative's wives to his. Obviously if this inheritor has HIV or another STI, the new wives stand a good chance of "inheriting" those diseases. Conversely, if he contracts such diseases from any of the dead relative's wives, he can pass them on to his wives. Widowhood rites are believed to be another contributing factor to the HIV/AIDS epidemic in Africa.

In Kenya and some other African countries, widows may be subjected to unwilling sexual encounters for "cleansing" purposes. In some villages in Kenya, selected men are paid to have sex with widows to cleanse them. Widows are required to sleep with such men, known as "cleansers", to be "cleansed" before they could attend the dead husband's funeral. Also, they must be "cleansed" in order to be inherited by their dead husband's brother or other male relative. Cleansers are believed to be spreading HIV in many villages in Kenya (Global Health Council, 2003). This custom is dangerous indeed but it evidently continues though it has always been unpopular among women.

REFERENCES

1. Armah, G. Ignorance on AIDS persists. *Daily Graphic*, April 4, 2001
2. Ardayfio, R. Gender inequality: a key factor in HIV/AIDS control. *Daily Graphic*, January 4, 2001.
3. Daileader, C (2001). Female genital mutilation: a woman's choice. *Global HealthLink*, 107: 9, 21.
4. Dawson, M.W. (1988). AIDS in Africa: historical roots. In N Miller and RC Rockwell (Eds). *AIDS in Africa: The Social and Policy Impact*, Lewiston/Queenston: Edwin Mellen.
5. Duh, S. V. (1991). *Blacks and AIDS: Causes and Origins*, Newbury Park: Sage Publications.
6. Duh, S. V. (1994). *Money Talks, Power Talks: The New World Disorder*, New York: Vantage Press.
7. Duh, S. V. (1999). *One More Time*, Accra: Ghana Universities Press.
8. Ghana Classified. Kufour meets British High Commissioner. Available at *www.ghanaclassified.com*. Accessed on 2/22/01.
9. Global Health Council (2003). Kenyan women reject sex "cleanser". Available at *www.globalhealth.org/news/article/3460/ newsletter*. Accessed on 25/8/03.
10. Green, E.C. et al (2001). We're talking about....*AIDSLink*, 65: 4

11. Hag, C (1988). Data on AIDS in Africa: an assessment. In N Miller and RC Rockwell (Eds). *AIDS in Africa: The Social and Policy Impact*, Lewiston/Queenston: Edwin Mellen.

12. Halperin, D (2001). Is poverty the root cause of African AIDS? *AIDSLink*, 65: 9.

13. Susser, J and Stein, Z (2000). Culture, sexuality and women's agency in prevention of HIV/AIDS in South Africa. *American Journal of Public Health*, 90: 1042-1048.

14. Tawfik, Y (2000). Promising interventions for improving private practitioner's practices in child survival. *Global HealthLink*, 105: 19-20.

15. UNAIDS. The interplay of factors driving the sexual transmission. Available at *www.unaids.org*. Accessed on 1 /29/01

16. Winkelstein, W et al (1987). Sexual practices and risk of infection by human immunodeficiency virus: the San Francisco Men's Study. *Journal of American Medical Assoc*, 257: 321-325.

CHAPTER SEVEN

THE CONSEQUENCES OF AFRICA'S BURNING

A factor whose presence can change wars, change the personalities of entire populations, disturb social life, give rise to new faiths, appreciably affect music, literature, and art cannot but be the vital concern of civilized man. Disease is such a factor. **—Henry Siegerist**

No disease in recent history has changed the personality of entire populations and disturbed social life the way AIDS has. In a relatively short period of time, this disease has done all the things Dr. Siegerist describes and more. As a pandemic, HIV/AIDS has touched every region of the world and affected people in all the ways described above. But nowhere has the effect been more extensive than the sub-Saharan African region. The devastation of Africa has been so ominous that the continent has aptly been described as being burnt.

In the last chapter, the fact that Africa is burning because of HIV/AIDS and why it is burning were extensively discussed. What then is the effect, the impact of this fire on the continent of Africa? Like a wild forest fire which can burn out of control if quick and appropriate action is not taken, the continent of Africa can "burn to the ground, to ashes" if aggressive and decisive measures are not taken to control the epidemic.

Unlike a forest fire that consumes vegetation, the fire of HIV/AIDS has the potential to decimate whole communities of people in sub-Saharan Africa. But this fire selectively consumes young and vibrant people in their most productive years of life. So in the process of taking down young people in the prime of their lives, the fire has the potential to destroy economies, health and educational systems, cause social upheaval, and destroy family structure. It is also a security threat with the potential of causing political instability, and some countries could collapse. Some of the consequences of the burning of Africa are tantamount to those of a war, and it requires the urgency of a war to control it.

Demographic Impact

The most radical demographic effect of the fire of HIV/AIDS is the reduction of life expectancy. Many countries in Africa had achieved remarkable improvements in their life expectancy in the post-independence era, but these achievements are being drastically eroded. Because HIV/AIDS affects African women disproportionately, other demographic effects are the lowering of fertility, creating of an excess of men over women, and the creating of millions of orphans (Knobel and VanLandingham, 2000; Brown, 2001).

Life expectancy is defined as the average number of years an individual is expected to live if current mortality trends continue to apply (Last, 1983). Life expectancy is different in different regions of the world and in different countries within regions. It is influenced by socio-economic conditions, cultural practices, health care infrastructure, and, to some extent, the genetic make-up of the people. According to the United Nations, Japan's life expectancy of 81 was the highest in the world in 2000, and with 43, Botswana had the lowest. In other words, a child born in the year 2000 in Japan was expected to live to be 81 years, whereas one born in Botswana was likely to live for only 43 years.

Life expectancy in most African countries was in the 40s in the early to middle part of the 20th century. After independence when these countries were being transformed from mostly agrarian to diversified industrial economies, life expectancy increased quite dramatically in many African countries. In some of these countries, life expectancy almost rivalled that of some developed countries. But HIV/AIDS has as dramatically been eroding these impressive gains. Ironically, the countries with the highest life expectancy in Africa were in the southern part of the continent prior to the HIV/AIDS epidemic; and countries in southern Africa are being hit the hardest by the epidemic. For example, life expectancy in Botswana that used to be 69 years without AIDS dropped to 43 by the year 2000; and in Zimbabwe, it is dropped to 44 years from 65 years. More importantly, these numbers are projected to worsen. By the year 2010, life expectancy is projected to drop to 33 years in Botswana, 35 years in Zimbabwe, and from 68 to 48 years in South Africa (Brown, 2001; UNAIDS, 2001).

Of course, low life expectancy means people are dying at a young age. So Africa is losing its young people in the millions. Each day nearly 6000 people are estimated to die in Africa from

AIDS. Since it takes 7-10 years from diagnosis to death, all 25.3 million people estimated to be living with HIV/AIDS in Africa are expected to die by the year 2010. In the year 2000, 2.4 million people died from AIDS; and by the end of 2000, Africa had buried more than 17 million HIV/AIDS victims, fully 75% of worldwide deaths (UNAIDS, 2001).

The hardest hit countries are going to lose the largest number of people. For example, Botswana is expected to lose almost 36% of its young adult population in 10 years. This is a huge blow to a country with the population of only about 1.5 million people. Other countries with high HIV/AIDS prevalence rates in southern Africa such as South Africa, Swaziland, Malawi, and Zimbabwe may lose nearly one-third of their young adults by 2010 (Brown, 2001). In South Africa alone, 6-10 million people are expected to die by 2010 (Stephenson, 2000). And in the eight African countries with at least 15% prevalence (all in southern Africa), about one-third of today's 15 year olds may be lost in the next 10 years (UNAIDS, 2000).

The situation in other parts of Africa is not as alarming as in southern Africa, but the trends there are also of concern. In East Africa Kenya, Ethiopia, Tanzania, and Uganda have HIV/AIDS prevalence rates of 8% to 14%. They are expected to lose those proportions of their population. West Africa is relatively less affected than East and southern Africa. However, Cote d'Ivoire is expected to lose more than 10% of its population; Nigeria had over 2.7 million people living with HIV/AIDS; and the crude death rate in Cameroon is expected to more than double by 2010 as a result of HIV/AIDS (UNAIDS, 2001).

Because AIDS claims the lives of people in their most fertile years of life, the demographic picture in many African countries is being affected by low fertility. This is particularly relevant in light of the fact that young adult females are three times and teenage girls are five times more likely than their male counterparts to be HIV-infected. Obviously the fewer females there are, the fewer babies would be born. As more females contract and die from HIV/AIDS, there is going to be an excess of males, and some of them might have to leave their native countries in order to get married (Brown, 2001).

With the foregoing discussion, it is obvious that the demographic landscape of Africa is changing and changing fast. With only 10% of the world's population, Africa is home to more than 70% of young adults living with HIV/AIDS worldwide. Since most, if not all of them, are expected to die in the next 10 years, Africa is going to lose a large portion of its young adults. In addition, 80% of children with HIV/AIDS in the world are in Africa. Again, these children are going to be lost. Furthermore, according to WHO data, the overall child mortality rate in Africa in 1999 was 15 per 1,000 live births; the global rate was 7 per 1,000, and that of Europe was 2 per 1,000 live births (American Public Health Assoc, 2001). But alas, there is a latent potential effect of HIV/AIDS on uninfected older adults.

Many people in their 60s and 70s in Africa depend on their grown children for economic survival. When the young adults are no longer available to provide for their older parents because of illness or death from HIV/AIDS, the older adults might be driven into destitution and earlier death (UNAIDS, 2001). Thus, the sum total effect of HIV/AIDS on the demography in Africa is a general shrinkage of the population. So to say that HIV/AIDS has the potential to decimate whole communities of people in Africa is no exaggeration.

Economic Impact

To say that a country's economy and prosperity depend on its people is almost too obvious a statement. The number of people in the workforce and the skills they possess are the engine that drives the country's economy. Without the technical know-how, resourcefulness, and hard work of a young and vibrant workforce, a country's prosperity, indeed its very survival may be in jeopardy. Many countries in Africa are in or headed for an economic jeopardy because of HIV/AIDS.

As stated in the last chapter, many countries in Africa have been marginalized economically because of wars, famine, economic mismanagement, and unfair trade practices. Most economies have depended quite heavily on agriculture, with the cultivation and exporting of cash crops. Others have been involved in the export of timber and minerals such as gold and diamond. There has been very little industrial activity in terms of manufactured goods, and most countries have depended on foreign countries for finished goods. Even countries like Nigeria and Angola with substantial oil reserves are still caught up in the process of exporting raw materials and importing finished goods.

The Republic of South Africa has been the exception to this phenomenon in sub-Saharan Africa. Blessed with abundant natural resources, South Africa has been the most industrialized country on the continent by harnessing its natural and human resources. However, the economic advantage in that country had not been enjoyed by all its citizens because of apartheid. With the demise of the apartheid system, South Africa became the jewel of black Africa. But just when it was freeing itself from the tentacles of apartheid, another monster with even longer tentacles was grabbing hold of the country.

Some other countries have achieved some measure of diversification. In southern Africa, Botswana, Zimbabwe, and Mozambique have been involved in some manufacturing and tourism. In West Africa, the Cote d'Ivoire has had a relatively stable and prosperous economy with a strong tourism industry. And in East Africa, the vibrant tourism industry in Kenya and Tanzania, mainly because of the Safaris, has been legendary. All these economies have depended upon a workforce of young people.

Many countries were already suffering from the shortage of a skilled workforce because of the brain drain phenomenon. In some countries, young people who would otherwise have been trained to join the workforce were fighting and dying in civil and territorial wars. Then the epidemic of HIV/AIDS reared it ugly head to make a rather bad situation worse, some would say hopelessly worse. The economic impact on the continent of Africa is daunting and promises to be even worse. According to the International Labour Organization, there is expected to be 11.5 million fewer people in the workforce by 2010, and in some countries the size of the workforce could be 35% smaller by 2020 (Ardayfio, 2000).

Africa, the poorest continent on earth, had been lagging behind others in economic growth. But small increases were going on and were due to expand with the dawn of the information age. However, a recent study by the World Bank painted a rather gloomy picture. The study found that income growth per capita in Africa was being reduced by about 0.7% per year because of HIV/AIDS. The income per capita would have grown at a rate of 1.1% per year in 1997-1999 had the prevalence rate of HIV/AIDS not reached 8.6°% in 1999. This would have been quite a respectable increase from the 0.4% per year growth observed in 1990-1997 (UNAIDS, 2001). The decline in per capita income growth, of course, is due to the shrinkage of the workforce due to HIV/AIDS and its attendant problems.

By the end of 2000, the prevalence of HIV/AIDS in sub-Saharan Africa was already 8.8%. That region also had the largest annual number of new cases. Most of the hardest hit countries did not have concrete plans in place to halt this trend. Therefore, the economic down turn appears to only get worse with time. Like the demographic impact, the economic consequences of HIV/AIDS are being felt the most by the hardest hit countries in southern Africa.

As stated above, South Africa has the largest economy in Africa. Per capita income there was six times the average for sub-Saharan Africa by the end of 2000. But with the largest number of cases of HIV/AIDS in the world, the economic impact on South Africa was the largest in the region. Studies have found that by 2010, the real gross domestic product (GDP) would be 17% lower than it would have been without the epidemic. In the

169

year 2001 terms, South Africa's economy would suffer a US$22 billion short fall. This US$22 billion short fall is more than twice the entire national production of any other country in sub-Saharan Africa with the exception of Nigeria (UNAIDS, 2001). Again, the shrinking workforce is contributing to this trend.

As employees become ill with HIV/AIDS, they leave their employment. This is particularly true with unskilled workers whose jobs often involve physical exertion. In South Africa, the HIV/AIDS prevalence is highest among the unskilled section of the workforce; likewise the unskilled have the highest unemployment rates—about 30%. In addition, there continues to be a shortage of skilled workers in most sectors of the economy, creating major impediments in business and production. Because of these factors, South Africa, whose national economy accounts for about 40% of the total economic output in sub-Saharan Africa, is likely to suffer 0.3% to 0.4% economic decline every year because of HIV/AIDS (UNAIDS, 2001).

The shortage of skilled workers is even more acute in Botswana; it is already importing skilled workers. With more people dying from AIDS, the unskilled labour pool is going to decline, and the unemployment rate among the unskilled is expected to fall by about 8%. Because of the diamond industry, the country's economy is more labour intensive than other economies in Africa. Therefore, with the decline in the workforce and resulting lower productivity, real GDP growth rate is expected to be slashed by about 1.5% per year. This would result in a dramatic 31% smaller economy by 2010 than it would have been without HIV/AIDS (UNAIDS, 2001).

The devastation of HIV/AIDS on the workforce in Africa has been taking a toll on companies. A study in South Africa in 1999 found more than 30% of mine workers and 26% of sugar mill workers were HIV-infected. About 90% of these workers were married and had an average of 6-7 dependants. The lost productivity from absenteeism, visit to company clinics, hospital admission, and cost of training replacement workers, cost the companies over US$1,000 per worker (UNAIDS, 2001). The number of employees lost to AIDS in South Africa in the next 10 years could account for about 50% of the current workforce in some South African companies (Stephenson, 2000).

Companies in the hardest hit countries in West and East Africa are similarly affected. In Cote d'lvoire, HIV/AIDS-related medical costs borne by four companies in Abidjan in 1993 was about US$1.8 to US$3.7 million. In 1997, the cost represented between 0.8% and 3.2% of the total wage bill. In Ethiopia, five firms were responsible for more than half of the burden of HIV/AIDS sickness in the mid-1990s. The burden was mostly in the form of increased absenteeism and medical care cost. And in a survey in Tanzania, the annual medical costs per employee incurred by six firms increased more than five-fold between 1993 and 1997, while burial costs to the companies increased more than five-fold (UNAIDS, 2001).

In light of the high costs of HIV/AIDS in terms of lost productivity, hiring and retraining, higher payments for insurance, and medical care, some companies are transferring some of their operations to countries less affected by the epidemic. Other companies are eliminating unskilled workers in an effort

171

to avoid paying benefits to those workers (UNAIDS, 2001). Obviously, this tactic deals a serious blow to the economic security of workers while shifting the responsibility for dealing with HIV/AIDS to families and the government.

As companies in the hardest hit countries find ways to protect their bottom line, the economic conditions of affected families are being adversely affected. Surveys have shown that when a family member suffers from HIV/AIDS, the household income is decreased. This is caused both by less money coming in, particularly if the sufferer is the main breadwinner, and increased medical care spending. When this happens, there are fewer purchases and diminished savings (UNAIDS, 2001). This in turn reduces the government's tax base, and the whole economy suffers. Indeed, the government suffers economic hardship for the same reasons as the private companies since the government is a major employer in many African countries. In this regard, certain infrastructural sectors of the government are being adversely affected as economies falter because of the HIV/AIDS epidemic.

The health sector.

The health sector in many African countries is being stretched quite thin. On a continent where health care expenditure in most countries has formed a rather small portion of the total budget, increases in the health budget have become necessary because of HIV/AIDS. For example, the governments' budget in health care sector is expected to be more than tripled in 10 years because of HIV/AIDS (UNAIDS, 2001). In some countries, the government's total budget is such that there is little room for any significant increases in the health budget. Therefore, to deal with the HIV/ AIDS crisis, other basic health care needs are being compromised (Brown, 2001).

In addition to the shortage of money for ministries of health, there is a shortage of manpower. Young adult workers who are more likely to acquire and die from HIV/AIDS include doctors, nurses, and other technicians who run hospitals and clinics. Furthermore, the health sector perhaps suffers more from the brain drain phenomenon than any other sector as doctors and nurses often find more lucrative employment overseas. Like mines and factories, the health care industry is losing some of its best-trained workers to HIV/AIDS. Since it takes quite a long time to train hospital workers, the health care industry is likely to starve for a long time to come. This is compounded by the fact that the total population of young adults continues to shrink, and the pool of people to be trained is simply not available in many countries. Those left to carry the burden of running the hospitals and clinics are getting very burned out (Stephenson, 2000). But in most hospitals in the hardest-hit countries, people with HIV/AIDS occupy the majority of beds.

The agricultural sector.

The agricultural sector is another area of the economy suffering from the HIV/AIDS epidemic. In most African countries, both cash crop and food production is mostly undertaken by small-scale farmers in rural communities. Families usually cultivate family owned land, and young adult members of the family usually do the bulk of the physical work. Also, families often hire day labourers to work on the farms both in planting and harvesting the crops. As families lose young adults to HIV/AIDS, the burden of maintaining the farms falls on the very young and older members of the family. Furthermore, the illness and death from HIV/AIDS drains the family's financial resources, leading to an inability to hire day labourers. And day labourers may not be readily available since that segment of the population tends to be among the hardest-hit by HIV/AIDS. The end result is the shortage of both cash crops and consumable foods.

The availability of consumable foods is particularly tenuous because of the involvement of women. In many countries, particularly among the rural populations, women are primarily responsible for the production of food crops for the family. Sometimes, they produce enough food for family consumption and for sale to supplement the family's income. According to the International Labour Organization, women produce between 60% and 80% of the continent's consumable food (Ardayfio, 2000). Since the epidemic is affecting women disproportionately in Africa, this important lifeline is being compromised, and both individual families and society as a whole suffer.

The effect of HIV/AIDS in the agricultural sector is having far-reaching consequences on the general economy and food security. For example, in West Africa, there have been reports of reduced cultivation of cash crops and food products. Reduced production of cotton in Burkina Faso and that of cocoa and coffee in Cote d'Ivoire have been observed. In Namibia, the problem is with livestock. As young adult males who tend to cattle herds contract and die from HIV/AIDS, the responsibility falls on women and children. Without the requisite experience to raise the cattle, the herd is often lost, with the potential to jeopardize the food security of those families and the country as a whole. In Kenya, young orphans who were farming in rural areas did not know where to go for information about food production. This is because in many countries including Namibia, Zimbabwe, and Malawi, agricultural extension workers, whose job it is to teach rural farmers about various farming techniques, were dying themselves from AIDS or spending a lot of time attending the funerals of AIDS victims (UNAIDS, 2001).

The education sector.

The education system is among the hardest hit sectors in terms of the number of both students and teachers. HIV-infected women tend to have fewer babies, and some die before they ever have a chance to bear children. Also, up to one-third of children born to these women would be infected, and they may die in 2-3 years after being born. Therefore, there is decreased number of children to go to school. In addition, in situations when both parents die from AIDS, the orphans tend to drop out of school either to earn money for survival or their caretakers could not afford school fees and other related costs. A study in Uganda found that the chance of an orphan going to school was halved when both parents died from AIDS (Brown, 2001; UNAIDS, 2001).

The HIV/AIDS epidemic also threatens the educational system by eroding the supply of teachers. Again, teachers tend to be in the 24-49 age group that is the most affected age group. In the hardest-hit countries such as Cote d'Ivoire, Central African

175

Republic, Zambia, and South Africa, the educational system is already being tasked; class size is increasing because of the shortage of teachers. In most of these countries, there are more teachers dying from AIDS than those being trained (Stephenson, 2000). For example, in Swaziland, it is estimated that twice as many new teachers need to be trained over the next 17 years just to keep up with their services at 1997 levels. In addition to sickness and death benefits, the cost of training and hiring new teachers is expected to be about US$233 million by 2016—more than the 1998-1999 total Swazi government budget for all goods and services (UNAIDS, 2001).

Perhaps the educational sector's demise is the most serious as far as the whole economy is concerned. Teachers are those who groom children from primary through tertiary levels to produce people with the skills and experience to service other sectors of the economy. So when the teachers are dying faster than could be trained to replace them, the whole economy suffers immensely. And when fewer children are attending school because children are dying from AIDS or being orphaned, the consequences are the same.

Family Structure

One of the most legendary, and perhaps the most sacred, institutions in African societies is family structure. It has been and continues to be the backbone of communities and nations. It has survived wars, coups d'etats, economic upheaval. It has survived colonial influences and modern foreign infiltration. In times of good and of bad, of plenty and of want, the African family has endured. But this legendary African institution is being threatened by HIV/AIDS in a way no other event has or, perhaps, can.

Most of the attention to HIV/AIDS has been directed at individuals; that is, the attention is directed at the management of those already infected and the prevention of the condition in uninfected individuals. But as discussed in the previous sections of this chapter, HIV/AIDS affects more than just the people infected. In contrast to most infectious diseases that mostly affect the very young and the very old, HIV/AIDS affects young adults. The condition, thus, affects the whole family emotionally, economically, socially, and physically during the long period of incapacitating illness (Knodel and vanLandingham, 2000). Thus as members of the family, if one is not *infected*, one may be *affected*. And when death ultimately occurs from AIDS, the family has to grapple with the problem of orphans.

When it comes to the effect of HIV/AIDS on the family, a lot of focus has been placed on the problem of AIDS orphans; that is, children who have lost one or both parents to AIDS. Obviously, the issue of orphanhood deserves a lot of attention, especially in Africa. By the end of 2000, AIDS had orphaned 13 million children under the age of 15 in Africa (Global Health Council, 2000). This figure is expected to reach 40 million by the year 2010 if current trends continue (Brown, 2001). If that happens, even the legendary resilience of the African family would be heavily taxed. To take care of that many orphans by the otherwise resilient extended family system of Africa would be very difficult, to say the least.

Like other problems with the HIV/AIDS epidemic, that of orphanhood affects some countries more than others. Thus, the countries in southern Africa that are hardest hit by the epidemic in general, are the most affected by the orphanhood problem. For example, South Africa, with the largest number of HIV/AIDS cases in the world, was estimated to have 800,000 orphans by the end of the year 2000 (Stephenson, 2000). Obviously, South Africa and other countries similarly affected have a mammoth problem on their hands. And if the projections are correct, this mammoth problem is going get much worse.

In most African countries, as it is in other developing countries, there is less public assistance for people affected by HIV/AIDS. Therefore, the responsibility for the care of AIDS orphans largely rests on the family. Since the family had already spent a lot on the care of the AIDS victim, it is often unable to provide adequately for the orphans. Therefore, many AIDS orphans risk dropping out of school, becoming street children, and being more susceptible to HIV infection through sexual abuse or becoming prostitutes by necessity. This is on top of having to cope with the stigma of having parents who died from AIDS (Stephenson, 2000; UNAIDS, 2001). Sometimes, when both parents die, very young teenagers may assume the responsibility of caring for younger siblings. Obviously, this situation is much less than desirable since these youngsters are themselves coping with the normal stresses of growing up.

As stated earlier, Africa faces the potential of more than 40 million children who might lose one or both parents to AIDS by 2010. Daunting as this problem is, I submit that it tells only half... or less...of the story. Whereas a lot of attention has been focused on the plight of children whose parents have died, other "AIDS orphans" have been overlooked. One tends to forget that when young adults die from AIDS, they leave behind their own parents who might be in their 50s, 60s, and 70s (Knodel and vanLandingham, 2000). In many cases, young adults are the main source of economic support for their parents in addition to that of their own children.

Unlike in Western societies where the (nuclear) family consists of the mother, father, and children, the extended family system prevails in Africa. Here the word *family* encompasses one's parents and other relatives in addition to one's spouse and children. When a person becomes successful, he or she is expected to support the whole "family". There is an Ashanti proverb which literally translates: "Your parents looked after you until your teeth came in, so you have to look after them until their teeth fall out." In other words, your parents ensured your survival from birth, when you were helpless, until adulthood; you have to ensure their survival in their old age, when they might be helpless, until their death. And many, if not most, successful young adults in Africa accept and take on this responsibility

Indeed, in most cases, the Ashanti proverb is not limited to one's parents; the successful person may take (financially) responsibility for parents, uncles and aunts, brothers and sisters, and nephews and nieces. Such a person (usually a young man) becomes what I call a "super father" (Duh and Willingham, 1987). So when such a person dies from AIDS, this economic lifeline is suddenly plugged, and many people are adversely affected. The super father tends to be the economic centre of the extended family, so when he dies from AIDS, the centre cannot hold, and things often do fall apart.

The destructive effect of HIV/AIDS on the family starts with the usual long debilitating illness, culminating in death. In most cases, when urban dwellers fall ill, they go to their hometowns to be taken care of by the family. Many family activities are altered in order to take care of the sick relative. For example, a study in the Cote d' Ivoire found that as a result of caring for HIV/AIDS patients, average family expenses were thus altered: outlay for school was halved; food consumption was decreased by 41% per capita; and health care expenditure was quadrupled (UNAIDS, 2001). Obviously, the whole family structure is disturbed by this one illness. With that kind of spending priority, everyone in the family suffers. And if the ill person is a super father type and dies, things do indeed fall apart in the family.

As stated earlier, the fact that Africa faces the potential of having about 40 million orphans by 2010 tells only half (or less) of the story. That 40 million represents children whose parents would have died from AIDS by 2010. That leaves another possible 40 million or more "orphans" if one assumes two living parents of the victim and other relatives as regards the super father syndrome. What would happen to the possible 80 million or more AIDS orphans by 2010? The immediate effect is that of the child orphans as discussed above. When adult orphans lose their lifeline, they often become destitute if there is no one else to fill the void. And the destitution, coupled with having to deal with the death of an adult child from a stigmatised disease, often leads to the early death of the older parents (UNAIDS, 2001). Ultimately, however, what is at stake is the very survival of the legendary African family structure. And as the family goes, so does the community, so does the nation.

The discussion in this chapter has been on some of the consequences of HIV/AIDS on the continent of Africa. The discussion has identified some adverse impacts that have taken place, currently happening, and the potential impact in the future. The consequences are in terms of life expectancy, general economy, health care, agriculture, education, and family structure. These topics are by no means exhaustive. Thus, it should be obvious that the epidemic is affecting almost every aspect of life on the continent. Since the consequences are negative, and in most cases quite drastic, it is not an exaggeration to state that Africa is burning. But some parts of the continent and some countries are burning more than others. In other words, some countries face a towering inferno, whereas others face a forest fire, and still others face a simmering under brush.

In some parts of the continent, whole communities are at the risk of being decimated. And in the case of Botswana, a whole country faces such a potential risk. At the current rate of new infections and deaths, the areas with wild fires face the potential of being burnt to the ground; and those simmering face the potential of becoming wild fires. Obviously, something has to be done and done quickly to put out these fires. What should be done to quench the fire of HIV/AIDS so it does not consume a whole continent? And who should do it? Before trying to answer these questions, I will discuss the general control of epidemics and that of HIV/AIDS in the next chapter.

REFERENCE

1. Ardayfio R. ILO launches programme against HIV/AIDS. *Daily Graphic,* December 8, 2000.

2. American Public Health Assoc. Child mortality rates decrease worldwide. *The Nations Health,* December 2000/January 2001; p. 15.

3. Brown L.R. (2001). Pandemic produces a missing generation, a population of orphans, a shortage of women. *AIDSLink,* 65: 6.

4. Duh, S. V. and Willingham, D. F. (1986). An ecological view of hypertension in blacks. *Journal National Medical Assoc.* 78: 617-619.

5. Global Health Council. Society for women and AIDS in Africa (SWAA) joins international partnership of organizations supporting children affected by HIV/AIDS. Available at www.globalhealth.org. Accessed on 10/21/2000.

6. Knobel, J and vanLandingham, M (2000). Children and older person: AIDS unseen victims. *American Journal of Public Health;* 90:1024-1025.

7. Last, J.M. (1983). *A Dictionary of Epidemiology.* New York: Oxford University Press.

8. Ntozi, J and Nakajiwas, S (1999). AIDS in Uganda: how has the household coped with the epidemic? In Orubuloye, IO et al (Eds) *The Continuing HIV/AIDS Epidemic in Africa: Response and Coping Strategies.* Canberra, Australia: Health Transition Centre, Australian National University; p. 155-180.

9. Stephenson, J (2000). AIDS in South Africa takes center stage. *Journal American Medical Assoc.*

10. UNAIDS (2001a). HIV/AIDS in Africa. Available at www.unaids.org. Accessed on 2/2/01.

11. UNAIDS (2001b). How does AIDS induce or deepen poverty? Available at www.unaids.org. Accessed on 31/24/01.

12. Zierler, S et al (2000). Economic deprivation and AIDS incidence in Massachusetts. *America Journal of Public Health;* 90: 1064-1073.

CHAPTER EIGHT

CONTROLLING THE HIV/AIDS EPIDEMIC

Since 1986, I have been "preaching" through my writings and speeches that the wrong approach has been taken to the control of the HIV/AIDS epidemic. Research and implementation programs have been primarily focused on medical therapy; that is, emphasis has been placed on drug and vaccine development. Very little attention has been paid to primary prevention, ignoring the fact that HIV/AIDS is a complex biological, social, and behavioural condition. But this approach to health care is not unique to the HIV/AIDS epidemic.

Throughout history human beings have approached illness with passive management on the part of the sick person. When people were ill in the olden days, they were given herbal preparations and other potions to treat the ailment (which still goes on to some extent); and with the advent of modern scientific medicine, sick people expect to be given a pill or an injection. Likewise, vaccination has been used to prevent and control many communicable diseases. Both treatment and prevention have, therefore, required little active participation with regard to individual responsibility to own health. So with the HIV/AIDS epidemic, people expected scientists to come up with a scientific solution in terms of a drug cure and vaccines. And the scientists accepted the challenge as exemplified by Dr. Lewis Thomas, a prominent American immunologist, in a 1988 essay: "...AIDS is a scientific research problem, to be solved *only by basic investigation in good laboratories....* (Italics added). {Thomas, 1988; p. 152).

The belief in science to solve the problem was reinforced by the impressive discoveries early in the epidemic: the causative agent was discovered in record time, and blood tests for antibodies to the virus were also quickly developed. Then the first antiretroviral medication (AZT) was discovered relatively quickly. These and other developments led people to assume that a cure and vaccine would be found soon. In the essay cited above, Dr. Thomas concluded: "The research done in the past few years has been elegant and highly productive, with results that tell us one thing: AIDS is a soluble problem, albeit an especially complex and difficult one... but the possibilities are abundant and the prospects are bright." (p. 152). Therefore, policy makers funnelled the bulk of resources to that end. They were also forced to go in that direction by the public in general and AIDS activists in particular who demanded a cure. To them, scientists could and must come up with a cure... and soon!

In this atmosphere, money flowed into research for drugs to cure HIV and treat other AIDS related illnesses. This led to a new level of entrepreneurial spirit as individual scientists and pharmaceutical companies competed against each other to find the elusive cure (Fee and Kreiger, 1993). The competition was not always friendly since major discoveries would lead to lucrative patents worth millions of dollars. In this regard, French researchers who were credited with co-discovering HIV accused their American co-discoverers of stealing from them. This led to the indictment of the head of the American group, Dr. Robert Gallo, who was later cleared of the charges. So with funding from government and other sources, and support, sometimes coercion, from the public, scientists have been working incessantly to find a cure for HIV.

As stated in earlier chapters, several drugs have been discovered since AZT, with the discovery of the protease inhibitors being hailed as a potential cure. But alas, after a few years of use, it became clear that the protease inhibitors, like the other drugs, were no cure for HIV. So as both scientific and popular media often announced the discovery of drugs with words like "promising" and "break through", people with HIV/AIDS had their hopes raised and dashed. And the HIV/AIDS victims and the rest of society have had similar ups and downs with regard to vaccine development.

Meanwhile, the social aspects of prevention have received little attention. Even if a cure or vaccine were to be discovered, behaviour modification would still be necessary for complete control of the epidemic. This fact is known to public health officials and other responsible entities, yet it has not succeeded in receiving the attention of policy makers. Therefore, as billions of dollars flowed to studies on cure and vaccine, few dollars became available for research on behavioural interventions. This state of affairs has prevailed throughout the history of the epidemic. For example, of the more than seven billion dollar U.S. government budget for HIV/AIDS for the year 2000, only 15% was allotted for education and prevention (Kelly, et al; 2000).

So what have been the consequences of the focus on a cure and vaccine? The simple answer is that it has failed since there is no cure or vaccine after more than 20 years of work. To be sure, the antiretroviral medications have reduced mortality and improved the quality of life for those HIV/AIDS patients who have access to them. But these medications have not dramatically altered the nature and course of the pandemic. For one thing, these medicines are not readily available to most of the about 95% of the people with HIV/AIDS worldwide who live in developing countries.

Even in countries where these medicines are available, not everyone there has access to them; and the epidemic picture there has not changed much. For example, in the United States, data from the CDC suggest that the number of people with HIV infection was slowly increasing at the end of 2000 because of sustained levels of HIV transmission. And the sustained level of transmission was due to high-risk sex and drug use behaviour in concert with increased survival among people who had received the antiretroviral medications. Other data showed increased high-risk behaviour among male homosexuals because they were less concerned about HIV diagnosis because of the availability of treatment (Fleming et al, 2000).

The foregoing discussion indicates that the focus on drug therapy and vaccine development has not had a demonstrable effect on slowing the HIV/AIDS pandemic. Indeed, the epidemic rages on, spreading in and consuming some populations like wildfire, partly because of this misplaced emphasis. Without a cure or vaccine, how is the war on HIV/AIDS going to be won? How should we approach the control of this devastating pandemic? The answer to these questions is both simple and complex. The simple answer is that we should rededicate our efforts to towards prevention, towards behaviour modification. But it is not that simple because human behaviour is a complex phenomenon. Before offering a complex answer, a review of the problems with drug therapy and vaccine development is in order.

Drug therapy.

The complexities involved with the development of a cure for HIV have been discussed in detail in Chapter Four. It has been made clear that a cure is not available and one was not on the horizon. Here are the main points regarding the numerous difficulties involved with coming up with a cure or even an effective treatment.

1. Like every virus, HIV has to live inside a host cell in order to survive. It is difficult, if not impossible, to get medicines inside the cell to kill the virus without killing the human cell. Therefore, all the medicines licensed to treat HIV by the end of 2000 worked by interfering with the reproductive cycle of HIV after it has entered the human cell, not an ideal way to effect a cure. Early research on medications that could block the virus from entering human cells demonstrated similar problems of side effects and resiatance to the earlier drugs.

2. The highly active antiretroviral therapies (HAART), which were

touted as cure when they first came out, are very difficult to take. They require individualized approach to therapy in terms of when to start medications, which combination of drugs is appropriate for a particular patient, if and when to stop the regimen for some time (drug holiday or pulse therapy), when to switch drugs if the initial combination is ineffective or no longer works. This requires access to clinicians who are experienced in treating HIV disease because studies have demonstrated that there is a strong association between access to experienced providers and better outcome (Levy et al, 2000).

3. HAART is a complex therapy which requires patients to take many pills (pill burden) at different times, some with food and others without food; and the patient has to deal with side effects which may be just a nuisance or very serious. The serious side effects range from lipodystrophy to kidney and liver failure to fatal mitochondrial dysfunction. All these have the tendency to tie the patient down with limited quality of life; that is, the therapy controls the patient.

4. The complex nature of HAART, particularly as regards side effects and lifestyle changes, makes it very difficult for most patients to take the drugs as directed. As stated in Chapter Four, at least 95% compliance is required to decrease viral load to below a level of detection. However, only 28% of patients have been found to achieve the requisite 95% level of compliance. And non-compliance often leads to the emergence of drug resistant viruses. Also, the virus frequently undergoes mutation leading to the emergence of drug resistant viruses. Drug resistance renders these medicines useless, carrying with it the additional danger of the transmission of drug-resistant viruses. Recall that drug resistant viruses have already been isolated in some parts of Africa where the use of these antiretroviral medications is not widespread.

5. Finally, the prohibitive cost of the medicines makes it impossible for them to reach all those who need them even in developed countries. In developing countries, they are largely out of reach to most individuals and many governments. Then there is the treatment of opportunistic infections and other conditions associated with HIV/AIDS such as depression and malnutrition. And when HAART therapy produces other diseases like diabetes and hyperlipidemia, then it almost requires that the patient be

independently wealthy to manage the disease with medical therapy.

The bottom line regarding antiretroviral therapy for the cure of HIV is that it is very expensive, difficult, and in some cases dangerous to take, and it is largely ineffective on a long-term basis because of its numerous problems. A lot of research has gone into finding the "perfect" drug to cure HIV, but none has been found; neither is there a real hope of finding one in the near future. The problems with finding a cure have largely been because of the complex nature of HIV.

In addition to the above facts, I have often taken a seemingly simplistic view in my speeches, particularly to legislators and other policy makers, on the issue of drug cure for HIV. First, I give a brief discussion on the microbiology of viruses and why it is difficult to have a drug go inside a cell to kill the virus without killing the cell. Then I add that, that is the reason why there is no cure for any viral disease. Members of the audience are often surprised to hear the last statement. Yes; no medicine has ever cured a viral disease in history. Most viral illnesses are self-limiting; that is, they do not cause any serious disease or they weaken the body to the extent that other organisms like bacteria cause serious disease or death. I conclude that scientists have been trying for more than a hundred years to find a cure for the common cold without success. If they cannot find a cure for the cold viruses, how can they find one for such a complex virus as HIV?

The comparison with the cold virus is for illustrative purposes only. It would be too simplistic and shallow-minded to conclude that just because scientists have been unable to find a cure for the common cold, they cannot find one for HIV. A more appropriate statement should be that finding a cure for HIV would very difficult, if not impossible, because of the nature of viral illnesses. The illustration is made to remind people that prevention is the most effective way of dealing with the control of the HIV/AIDS epidemic. Therefore, as much or more resources should be directed at prevention as cure efforts. Certainly, research on finding a cure should proceed but it should not be at the neglect of prevention.

Vaccine development.

The search for a vaccine against HIV has encountered peaks and valleys similar to that for a cure. In fact, it has encountered mostly valleys, and most of the peaks have actually been bumps. Thus, with hundreds of scientists all over the world spending millions of dollars and hours, there has not been a vaccine, nor is there likely to be one in the near future. Several obstacles have contributed to this state of affairs, relating mostly to the complex nature of HIV.

The principle behind vaccine development is based upon the human body's ability to "remember" encounters with infectious agents. This is why when we get infectious diseases such as chicken pox, we may be protected for life from that disease. For example, when we are infected with chicken pox, the body makes many antibodies and generates other immune cells to fight off the infection. With recovery from the illness, surplus antibodies remain in the body for life so that any time chicken pox viruses enter the body, they are destroyed quickly before they can cause illness.

A vaccine is made out of a form of an organism that has been rendered harmless and is introduced into the body to prime it to fight off a particular disease. That is, when we are given the vaccine, the body perceives the harmless organism as real and makes antibodies and other immune cells to destroy it. This is termed *immune response*. The surplus antibodies remain in the body, and if the real organism enters the body at a later date, it is quickly destroyed by the antibodies before it can cause disease.

The simple rule about vaccine development is that the vaccine should be capable of mounting an immune response without causing disease. To be sure a vaccine does not cause disease, the organism is weakened or a derivative of the organism is used in the preparation of the vaccine. In this regard, a vaccine could be made from live attenuated virus as in measles vaccine, killed virus as in polio (Salk) vaccine, or from a subunit derivative as in hepatitis B vaccine. Of the three types of vaccine, the one made from the live attenuated organism is the most immunogenic; that is, it is the most protective, and one administration is often protective for life.

The paradox of live attenuated virus vaccine is that it is the most immunogenic because such a vaccination is the closest to natural infection. However, it is also the most dangerous because it can sometimes cause the disease it is supposed to prevent. For example, a few children who received the oral polio (Sabine) vaccine, prepared from live attenuated polioviruses, developed polio annually from the vaccination. The small risk for paralytic polio was accepted by scientists and the general public perhaps because polio is not universally fatal, though it can kill its victims.

But in the year 2000, the CDC and American Academy of Paediatrics recommended against the use of the oral vaccine because of the risk of acquiring polio from the vaccine.

Obviously, the most effective potential vaccine against HIV would be the one made from the live virus. But because HIV infection would most likely lead to death, it is almost unthinkable to embark on the development of an AIDS vaccine from the live virus. Scientists are even apprehensive about using the killed virus because of the fear that once the vaccine has been administered, the virus might somehow wake up and cause HIV infection.

From the foregoing discussion about live attenuated and killed virus vaccines, it should be obvious why most of the work on finding a vaccine for HIV/AIDS has been concentrated on the subunit process. The subunit process is not without problems. The main one is that the component of the virus isolated for vaccination should usually be carried on a whole molecule called a vector before it can mount an immune response. The vector could be a synthetic molecule or another (less dangerous) organism. The vector-subunit complex should be precise enough to mount an immune response in addition to being practical for vaccination.

The use of vaccination to control the HIV/AIDS epidemic involves two types of vaccines—a therapeutic vaccine and a preventive vaccine. The therapeutic vaccine is for people with HIV infection. The antibodies the body develops from the vaccine would neutralize HIV already present in the body and destroy future viruses the patient might acquire. The preventive vaccine is for people who have not been exposed to HIV, and its purpose is as discussed above.

The first HIV/AIDS vaccine using the subunit process was developed by a team of French scientists headed by Daniel Zagury. The vaccine consisted of purified gp160 subunit of HIV with killed vaccinia (smallpox) virus as the vector. Zagury inoculated himself with the vaccine in November 1986, and then he tested it in human volunteers in Zaire. The vaccine produced immune response in some of the volunteers, but the process of inoculation was too complicated for it to be feasible as a useful vaccine (Matthew & Bolognesi, 1988).

The first AIDS vaccine to undergo testing in the United States also employed a gp160 subunit but the vector used was the household chemical alum. The trials were conducted in October 1987 by the National Institutes of Health (NIH). Initial results were ambiguous but the researchers believed that increasing the dose levels might improve the vaccine's performance. Also in 1987, a vaccine using another subunit of HIV called gp120 underwent trials in Switzerland with similar unimpressive results (Matthews & Bolognesi, 1988). Subsequent work on vaccine development in different parts of the world has employed variations of the earlier work by the Zagury group and the NIH. Scientists have been working incessantly to improve upon the earlier work.

Like the search a cure for HIV/AIDS, the search for a near perfect vaccine has been frustrating, again because of the complex nature of HIV. The difficulty in developing an effective vaccine is three-fold: (1) finding an effective and safe vaccine, (2) performing human trials on a mass scale, and (3) overcoming liability problems.

To be effective and safe, the potential vaccine should produce an immune response without causing the disease or other intolerable side effects. But it is not enough to just produce an immune response; the immune cells must also be able to destroy HIV, and that is what the main problem has been. It appears that most of the vaccines tested so far have produced an immune response, but HIV infected patients given the trial vaccines went on to develop AIDS. That means the antibodies and other immune cells produced were not able to destroy HIV. This is not too surprising because the natural HIV infection produces immune response, but the antibodies produced do not seem to be able to destroy the virus.

Another problem with vaccine development is the fact that there are so many strains or subtypes of HIV. Even if a vaccine were developed which could mount an immune response and neutralize HIV, it might not work for other strains of the virus. For example, Subtypes A and D are more common in East Africa, whereas subtype C in predominant in southern Africa, and the predominant subtypes in West Africa are A and a combination of A/G virus. And the predominant virus in the United States and Europe is subtype B. Interestingly, most of the research on vaccine development has been with the subtype B virus, not with the subtypes found in Africa where more than 70% HIV/AIDS prevalence worldwide is.

The second problem involves logistics and ethics. Since HIV/AIDS is a pandemic, and particularly when there are so many strains of HIV, a potential vaccine should be tested in millions of people in different geographic areas. It would be a logistical nightmare to recruit that many people and get vaccine material and equipment to all of them. The ethics of the issue is the selection of people to receive a test vaccine. Getting volunteers for therapeutic vaccines would not be too difficult since people with HIV infection have little to lose by receiving a vaccine. Preventive vaccine is a different matter. It necessarily has to be given to healthy people, those without HIV infection. Since HIV infection will most likely end in death, it is unlikely that millions of people would volunteer when it cannot be guaranteed that the vaccine would not cause infection. In this regard, how to get uneducated people to sign informed consent is a big dilemma. Then there is politics.

During the international conference on AIDS in Africa in Tanzania in 1988, Dr. Robert Gallo of the U.S. National Cancer Institute appealed to the Tanzanian health minister to permit large scale vaccine trials in Tanzania and other central African countries. Gallo's suggestion was regarded as racist, and officials of those countries did not embrace the idea (Duh, 1991). Also at issue politically is the ownership of vaccines. In 1993, the U.S. National Institutes of Health (NIH) planned a multi-candidate trial of therapeutic vaccines. It wanted the vaccines to be donated by the companies that manufactured them. Four of the manufacturers agreed but the fifth one, MicroGeneSys, refused to donate its vaccine. The trial had to be suspended. Speaking on the issue at the 9th International Conference on AIDS in Berlin, Dr. Anthony Fauci of the NIH said: "If the companies do not donate the vaccine, it will be very difficult, if not impossible, to conduct the trial using multiple vaccines." (American Health

Consultants, 1994; p.103). Also, in the year 2000, collaboration between Kenyan and British scientists on vaccine development went sour when the British scientists decided to go it alone in testing a candidate vaccine and obtaining a patent for it.

The liability problem is one of the toughest facing vaccine developers. From the earliest days of vaccine development work, there has been the fear of lawsuits if any vaccine was found to cause harm. And there is evidence that the fear of litigation has slowed the progress on vaccine development. Some manufacturers have been afraid to test promising vaccines on a mass scale; others have simply stopped work on HIV vaccines (Cohen, 1992). The fear of litigation is based upon the fact that since the potential vaccine might not be 100% effective, people who get HIV infection after receiving the vaccine might sue the manufacturer. The manufacturer would suffer financial losses whether or not it could be proved that the vaccine actually caused the infection.

To use a vaccine as the major tool of controlling the epidemic will require the development of a near perfect vaccine. Such a vaccine would ideally require a single dose, be given orally, cover all strains of HIV, have little or no side effect, last for a lifetime, not require refrigeration, and be cheap enough for developing countries to afford it. Obviously it would be extremely difficult to develop such a vaccine. Then there is the need to recruit and train thousands of workers to administer the vaccine. For preventive vaccine, how would it be decided whom to vaccinate? Would everyone be vaccinated or would the vaccine be given to people in so called risk groups? If it is limited to risk groups, how would such groups be identified? (Henderson, 2000).

Despite the formidable problems facing vaccine development, work has been going on all over the world to find one. In this regard, the International AIDS Vaccine Initiative (IAVI) was formed in 1996 with the purpose of allowing scientists to share ideas and support each other's efforts in vaccine development. Also, as an organization, IAVI would be more able to raise funds than individual scientists could. The focus of IAVI has been to develop several vaccines for different strains of HIV, rather than finding a single vaccine to be used everywhere in the world.

In July, 2000 IAVI unveiled its "Scientific Blueprint 2000: Accelerating Global Efforts in AIDS Vaccine Development". The aim of the blueprint was to develop an effective vaccine in the shortest possible time by widening the vaccine pipeline. It called for putting 25 innovative vaccine designs into development and conducting head-to-head trials among them with the hope of leading to six to eight efficacy trials by the year 2007. The new plan was expected to slash the time needed between a product's design and global licensure by as much as 50% (Henderson, 2000).

The Scientific Blueprint 2000 also called for greater focus on vaccines for use in developing countries. This is because only a few of the vaccines in development were tailored for use in developing countries where over 95% of HIV/AIDS cases and new infections were. In this regard, IAVI announced during the XIII International AIDS Conference in South Africa that Medicines Control Agency of Britain had approved a Phase I testing of a DNA vaccine based on HIV subtype A, the most common strain found in Kenya and some others parts of Africa. The trial would involve 18 volunteers in Oxford, England, with another trial in

Nairobi, Kenya, three to six months later. Though more than 25 vaccines had been tested in humans so far, this is the first one designed for Africa (Henderson, 2000).

Researchers were quite optimistic that the new blueprint would help in developing a usable vaccine within the next ten years. But that optimism is tempered by the fact that for more than 15 years since HIV was identified as the cause of AIDS, only one vaccine strategy had progressed to Phase III efficacy trials by the year 2000. The report, thus, proposed parallel, rather than sequential, Phase III efficacy trials in several countries or regions hardest hit by HIV/AIDS. This was to accelerate the testing process, in addition to determining the extent of protection by each vaccine design in order to avoid delays in licensing and implementing use of the vaccines in different populations (Henderson, 2000).

Where Do We Go From Here?

The discussion so far in this chapter has summarized where we have been as far as the HIV/AIDS pandemic goes. It has been made clear that emphasis has been wrongly placed. We seem to have forgotten that HIV/AIDS is not just a disease; it is an epidemic, a pandemic. An epidemic cannot be controlled without stopping the occurrence of new cases. This has been the approach to epidemics and disease outbreaks such as cholera, measles and hepatitis A. Major epidemics and other disease outbreaks in history have all been controlled by stopping new cases through epidemiologic means.

A lot of the knowledge on HIV/AIDS has been obtained from epidemiological studies. Indeed, epidemiology is indispensable to the understanding of a new disease, particularly one with a pandemic distribution of HIV/AIDS. The use of epidemiology has led to the understanding and better control of many diseases in history

Epidemiology may be defined as the study of the *distribution* and *determinants* of diseases and injuries in human populations. The way diseases are distributed and the factors that influence the distribution (determinants) can lead to intelligent guesses about the nature of a particular disease. The implication from the definition of epidemiology is that diseases are unevenly distributed in populations, and the uneven distribution can be a basis for concluding causal relationships between certain population characteristics and diseases. Morris (1955, p. 395) put it this way:

> The main function of epidemiology is to discover groups in the population with high rates and with low, so that causes of disease and of freedom from disease can be postulated.... The biggest promise of this method lies in relating disease to ways of living of different groups. And by doing so to unravel "causes" of disease about which it is possible to do something.

The significance of the above quotation is the use of epidemiological studies to find causes of disease about which something could be done. The implication here is that there may not be a need to find the true "scientific" cause of a disease or an epidemic in order to control it. Modification of certain factors that influence the cause and/or course of the disease may lead to adequate or even complete control of a disease. A classic example of this phenomenon is John Snow and the water pumps involved in a cholera epidemic in London.

An outbreak of cholera was killing hundreds of people in London in 1853. As scientists struggled to find the cause of the epidemic and ways to control it, John Snow, a London physician, made a simple suggestion—turn off the water pumps supplying water to the neighbourhoods with the highest numbers of deaths from cholera. This was done, and the epidemic was brought under control. The epidemic was controlled without knowing the cause of cholera. Dr. Snow accomplished his feat about 30 years before Koch discovered *Vibro cholera* as the causative agent of cholera (Duh, 1991).

Snow used epidemiological principles to study the cholera epidemic and came to the conclusion that cholera might be transmitted by discharge of faecal material into water supplies. He investigated the water supply for each household where a fatal cholera attack had occurred. His figures demonstrated that most deaths were occurring in the neighbourhoods supplied by one company, the Southwark and Vauxhall Company. The lowest number of deaths was in areas supplied by another company, the Lambeth Company. It turned out that the Southwark and Vauxhall Company drew its water from the Thames River downstream where the water had been contaminated by human waste. The Lambeth Company drew water upstream where the water was free of contamination. Snow's analysis of death rates showed a 20:1 ratio between areas supplied by the two companies; that is, individuals living in households supplied by the Southwark and Vauxhall Company (contaminated water) were dying 20 times more frequently than those supplied by the Lambeth Company.

The significance of the Snow story is the fact that Dr. Snow focused his attention on the aspects of the epidemic *about which something could be done*. Something was done based on his findings, and the epidemic was controlled—30 years before the causative agent of cholera was discovered! It is interesting to note that, with the knowledge of the causative agent and effective antibiotics to treat it, personal hygiene (originating from Snow's idea) is still the recommended approach to controlling cholera infections and epidemics. Washing hands meticulously, boiling water before drinking or using it to prepare food, and controlling flies are extremely effective in controlling cholera transmission even today. These measures do not require the knowledge of the causative agent or the pathogenesis of cholera. In addition, they are more practical, simpler, and cheaper to implement.

I have recounted the story about John Snow and the cholera epidemic to make a point, which is that we need to apply more epidemiology to the control of the HIV/AIDS epidemic. We should do this by applying Morris's definition of epidemiology; that is, trying to focus more attention on the aspects of HIV/AIDS about which something can be done (Duh, 1991). We should bear in mind that using epidemiological principles to develop and implement prevention programs is simpler, cheaper, and does not carry with it side effects as drug and vaccines can.

It is sad that the world missed the opportunity to have the AIDS epidemic under control. We have known from the beginning of the epidemic how to control it, but we have not taken full advantage of that knowledge. That is, even before HIV was discovered, epidemiologists had outlined the means of transmission. All we had to do was reverse or modify the activities that promoted transmission, and the epidemic would have been under control. It did not require the discovery of the causative agent. Had we focused more on that aspect, the pandemic would have peaked and, perhaps, the prevalence would have decreased. Indeed, the HIV infection incidence peaked in the United States during the mid-1980s because of successful prevention strategies such as blood screening and donor deferral, counseling and testing programs, and behaviour risk reduction through education (Fleming et al, 2000). But as soon as HIV was discovered, we directed almost all our efforts to the virus in trying to find a drug and vaccine against it.

Without a doubt, knowing the causative agent of AIDS is important in the overall approach to the control of the epidemic. But we seem to have overlooked the obvious; that is, it is better to prevent transmission than to try to control the virus with drugs and vaccines. Pre-transmission prevention is certainly more effective, cheaper, and safer than post-transmission management. For example, it costs relatively little to screen donated blood for HIV antibodies. This process has effectively rendered HIV transmission through blood transfusion almost a thing of the past in most countries. Similarly, it costs a lot less to supply drug addicts with clean needles or counsel people on sexual abstinence and supply them with condoms.

Studies have demonstrated that given enough information and the appropriate empowerment, people can and do change their behaviour. For example, studies have shown a correlation between the amount of HIV/AIDS education and sexual behaviour among high school students. That is, those who received the most intensive HIV/AIDS and sex education showed the greatest decrease in frequency of unprotected sexual intercourse, multiple sexual partnerships, and the greatest increase in condom use (Ku et al, 1992, Holtzman et al, 1994). Similar results have been observed among university students (Cochran et al, 1990; Strauss et al, 1992). Drug users have similarly been educated to change their behaviour with regard to needle sharing and sexual activity (Kall et al, 1990; McCusker et al, 1992); and the behaviour change resulted in decreased incidence of HIV transmission (Des Jarlais et al, 1994). These reports are from the United States, several European countries, and Thailand. In the case of Thailand, impressive reductions in HIV/AIDS prevalence among commercial sex workers have been achieved through aggressive counseling and 100% condom availability programs, and a nationwide epidemic was stopped in its tracks (Global Health Council, 2001). In Africa, Uganda has become a model for the rest of the continent and the world for its prevention programmes which have brought about a reduction in prevalence from 14% in 1998 to 8% by 2000. This impressive accomplishment in Uganda was through aggressive campaign on prevention, not the use of drugs or vaccine. And Senegal stopped HIV/AIDS early before it could explode into an epidemic in that country (UNAIDS, 2000).

These pre-transmission programs have not been widely applied because of the misconception that drug users are unwilling or unable to change their behaviour (Chitwood, 1994). Likewise, it has been suggested that sexuality is biologically based and socially sanctioned, and young people in particular cannot change their sexual behaviour (Fineberg, 1988). Without a doubt, behaviour change is very difficult, but it is not impossible as illustrated by the above-cited and other studies. Therefore, in the absence of effective treatment and vaccines, programs to effect behaviour change must be established, expanded, and maintained if we are serious about controlling the HIV/AIDS pandemic.

The goal of controlling an epidemic is twofold: (1) to improve the health status of people with the ill condition, and (2) to keep those without the condition from acquiring it. And the best approach to both is prevention (Duh, 1991). Since there is no cure or vaccine and none likely in the near future, I submit that prevention should be the approach to controlling the HIV/AIDS epidemic.

There are three levels of prevention—primary, secondary, and tertiary. Primary prevention is to ensure that healthy people are not exposed to the causative agent of a disease. Once people acquire the causative agent, secondary prevention ensures that they do not progress to the disease stage. Tertiary prevention effects rehabilitation and improvement in health status after the disease stage has been reached. For the HIV/AIDS epidemic, we should employ primary prevention to ensure that people not exposed to HIV remain free of exposure, secondary prevention to ensure that those with HIV infection do not progress quickly to AIDS, and tertiary prevention to ensure that AIDS patients live as long and healthful lives as possible (Duh, 1991). We should do away with our obsession with finding a cure.

To state that we should do away with our obsession with finding a cure does not mean we should leave people with HIV disease to die. They can be managed, short of a complete cure, such that they can maintain a relatively healthful existence. The goal should be to significantly improve upon the very short life span of many AIDS patients, as it currently exists. After all, there are many incurable diseases, and we seem satisfied just to treat such diseases instead of cure them. There is no cure for genetic diseases like cystic fibrosis and sickle cell anaemia, but victims of those diseases are given various treatments that permit them to have a reasonably long life span. There is no cure for hypertension, diabetes, asthma and arthritis, but their victims have a normal life span with appropriate treatment. Why can't we do the same for people with HIV disease?

Management of HIV Disease.

It should be remembered that people do not die directly from the AIDS virus. The virus destroys the immune system, and then the victims acquire infections (opportunistic infections) from other organisms from which they die. Theoretically, if an HIV infected person were completely protected from infectious agents, he or she could live a normal life span. Obviously, it is impossible to protect from infectious agents under ordinary living conditions since the natural environment is full of all kinds of harmful organisms. Since it is impossible to eliminate the risk of infection, the goal should be to reduce the risk as much as possible. Therefore, the approach to HIV disease should be that of screening, early detection, and treatment. This approach, of course, constitutes secondary and tertiary prevention.

Screening is the key to secondary prevention. It involves taking careful history to determine who are likely to acquire HIV and doing HIV antibody testing to diagnose HIV infection. People with HIV infection should be quickly started on a treatment program. Treatment does not necessarily have to involve antiretroviral medications; its objective is to delay as much as possible the progression to AIDS. Thus, activities to maximize the immune status should be pursued; that is, counseling on proper nutrition, exercise, stress management, and prevention and treatment of cofactor diseases such as syphilis, chancroid, herpes, and other STIs. All patients diagnosed with HIV infection should undergo tuberculin skin testing, and those testing positive should receive anti-tuberculosis prophylactic medication. Judicious use of antiretroviral medications should be considered for patients under appropriate conditions. Initial CD4 count should be recorded at the time of diagnosis and monitored frequently.

Once the CD4 level reaches below 200, the person is considered to have AIDS regardless of whether or not AIDS defining symptoms are present. Closer clinical monitoring should then be instituted. All AIDS patients should be considered for PCP (*pneumocystis carinii* pneumonia) and Candidiasis prophylaxis. They should stay away from sick people and other situations where contact to communicable diseases is likely. People with weight lose should be considered for appetite enhancer medications such as Megestrol, Cyproheptadine (Periactin), and Dronabinol (Marinol). They should be offered nutritional supplements to boost their weight. These measures would prevent the development of opportunistic infections or at least delay it. But when opportunistic infections do occur, they should be treated quickly and aggressively. In this regard, research should focus on finding effective drugs for the numerous opportunistic organisms and other AIDS-defining diseases.

With the combination of secondary and tertiary prevention as outlined above, people with HIV disease could have a relatively normal existence. The key is early detection and aggressive management. Thus, a lot more resource should go into screening programs so that people with HIV disease would get to early treatment. This approach is certainly cheaper and should be more effective than trying to cure the virus.

Primary prevention of HIV infection.

The purpose of primary prevention is to avoid the acquisition of HIV. In this regard, the means and modes of transmission as discussed in Chapter Three should be the focus of prevention programs. That is, ways to educate people about avoiding sexual transmission, needle sharing in drug use, mother-to-child transmission, and transmission through breast-feeding should be explored. Of particular importance is the consideration of individual and group characteristics such as cultural and religious beliefs and practices. As regards sexual and drug use education, the goal is to effect behaviour modification. However, behaviour modification should not be limited to people whose behaviour may place them at risk for infection but should include family members, legislators, other policy makers, and members of the media (Fee and Krieger, 1993).

Policy makers and the media play a critical role directly or indirectly in the control of the HIV/AIDS epidemic. However, some of them have been a hindrance to the dissemination of health education messages. For example, laws have been passed to prevent the discussion of sexual matters in schools and prohibit the distribution of clean needles to drug addicts. And the media have often refused to discuss sexual (educational) matters or advertise condoms. Paradoxically, both television and the print media often depict explicit sexual scenes. Thus, policy makers and members of the media should be educated to modify their behaviour by overcoming their individual and group inhibitions so as to make decisions based on scientific evidence (Fee and Krieger, 1993).

The ultimate aim of HIV/AIDS education is to affect population and individual characteristics through behaviour modification. Therefore, people should be empowered to change those behaviours that place them at risk for HIV infection. They should be provided with accurate, up-to-date, and understandable information on HIV transmission and how to prevent it. And the necessary tools should be provided or made available to them.

Sex education should include the frank discussion of human sexuality in the context of disease prevention. Individual responsibility should be stressed; that is, people should know that there is no cure or vaccine, and they are responsible for their own health vis-à-vis HIV/AIDS. In formal settings like schools and universities, AIDS education may be part of a comprehensive curriculum dealing with other STIs, unwanted pregnancy, drug and alcohol use, cigarette smoking, poor nutrition, and lack of exercise. Abstinence from these bad behaviours should be the focus; but the proper and consistent use of condoms should be discussed (Duh, 1991).

In addition to counseling against drug use in nonusers, drug users should be counseled against needle sharing. Obviously, the ideal situation is to get drug users to stop using drugs altogether. However, since most drug users are addicted to the drugs and only few treatment facilities are available for detoxification, providing addicts with clean needles is a prudent course. As mentioned earlier, studies have shown that supplying clean needles does not perpetuate drug use, and it does prevent the spread of HIV infection.

The main discussion in this chapter has been that no cure or vaccine for HIV/AIDS is forthcoming, that we have wasted a lot of time and resource on finding them, that we should redirect our efforts towards prevention programs. The HIV/AIDS epidemic can be controlled through primary, secondary, and tertiary prevention...if only we would do what is necessary in the sphere of prevention.

Prevention activities have proved to be effective when applied diligently. For example, the combination of decreased sexual activity and judicious use of condoms in the homosexual community was largely responsible for the slowing of the epidemic in that community. And the change in behaviour was due to the aggressive and effective education by members of that community. Likewise, education on needle sharing and needle exchange programs has had a positive effect on the epidemic in some countries. These successful programs should be emulated, built upon, and expanded to become the main stay of controlling the AIDS epidemic.

Many countries "saw the light" regarding the limits of drug cures and vaccines and have emphasized prevention. Indeed control activities in most African countries have been almost exclusively prevention. This is also due to an inability of these countries to afford the expense of drug therapies. Ironically, some have viewed this as a negative. For example, a group of researchers has decried the fact that international agencies, including United Nations and WHO, have emphasized prevention in Africa at the neglect of drug therapies (De Cock et al, 1993). They suggested that similar clinical studies to those that were going on in United States and Europe should be conducted in Africa to take care of Africans with AIDS. They concluded: "If we do nothing to address the requirements of care as the epidemic in Africa progresses, we will be justifiably criticized for having shown great interest in the study of AIDS in Africa but little interest in Africans who have AIDS" (De Cock *et al*, 1993 p. 1388).

I agree with De cock *et al* that something has to be done to take care of Africans with AIDS, but I disagree that the emphasis should be on antiretroviral therapy. The approach to HIV/AIDS in Africa should be the same as everywhere else—secondary and tertiary prevention for HIV/AIDS patients, and primary prevention to reduce the alarming rates of new infections going on in the continent.

The time has come to be bold and imaginative in our approach to the HIV/AIDS epidemic. The time has come to use the available resources wisely, to spread them out so that all populations get their fair share because HIV/AIDS is a global problem. The time has come to fund prevention programs equitably. We should stop our obsession with spending so much money on drug and vaccine development at the neglect of prevention. We should stop our obsession with trying to find a drug cure for HIV/AIDS because we already have a cure—prevention. Let us use it everywhere, and, in particular, in Africa so that the continent does not "burn to ashes". We can save Africa from HIV/AIDS!

REFERENCES

1. American Health Consultants (1994). Company refuses to donate vaccine for efficacy trial. *AIDS Alert*; 8: 103-105.
2. Auerbach, J.D. and Coates, T.J. (2000). HIV prevention research: accomplishments and challenges for the third decade of AIDS. *American Journal of Public Health;* 90: 1029-1036.
3. Cochran, S.D. et al (1990). Sexually transmitted diseases and acquired immunodeficiency syndrome (AIDS): changes in risk reduction behaviour among young adults. *Sexually Transmitted Diseases*; 17: 80-86.
4. Cohen, J (1992). Is liability slowing AIDS vaccine? *Science*; 256: 168 170.
5. De Cock, K.M et al (1993). Clinical research, prophylaxis, therapy, and care for HIV disease. *American Journal of Public Health*; 83: 1385 1389.
6. Des Jarlais, D.C. et al (1994). AIDS risk reduction and reduced HIV sero-conversion among injecting drug users in Bangkok. *American Journal of Public Health;* 84: 452-453.
7. Duh, S. V (1991). *Black and AIDS: Causes and Origins.* Newbury Park, Sage Publications.
8. Fee, E and Krieger, N. (1993). Understanding AIDS: historical interpretation and limits of biomedical individualism. *American Journal of Public Health*; 83: 1477-1486.
9. Fleming, P.L. et al (1998). Declines in AIDS incidence and deaths in the USA: a signal change in the epidemic. *AIDS*; 12: S55-561.

10. Fleming, P.L. et al (2000). Tracking the HIV epidemic: current issues, future challenges. *American Journal of Public Health* 90: 1037-1041.

11. Fineberg, H (1988). The social dimensions of AIDS. *Science*; 259: 128.

12. Global Health Council (2001). Strategic priorities essential to confronting the changing face of AIDS in Thailand. *AIDSLink*; 65:10

13. Henderson, C.W. (2000). First vaccine design for Africa cleared for testing in humans. *AIDS Weekly*; July 24, 2000: p. 2-3.

14. Holtzman, D et al (1994). Changes in HIV-related information source, instruction, knowledge, and behaviour among U. S. high school students, 1989 and 1990. *American Journal Public Health;* 84: 388-393.

15. Kall, K and Olin, R (1990). HIV status and changes in risk behaviour among drug users in Stockholm, 1987-1988. *AIDS*; 4: 153-157.

16. K elley, J. A. et al (2000). Bridging the gap between the science and service of HIV prevention: transferring effective research-based HIV prevention intervention to community AIDS service providers. *American Journal of Public Health*; 90: 1082 1089.

17. Ku, L.C. et al (1992). The association of AIDS education and sex education with sexual behaviour and condom use among teenage men. *Family Planning Perspective*; 24: 100-106.

18. Levi, J (2000). The public health challenge of the HIV epidemic. *American Journal of Public Health;* 90:1023-1024.

19. McCusker, J et al (1992). AIDS education for drug users: evaluation of short-term effectiveness. *American Journal of Public Health*; 82: 533-539.

20. Straus. P et al (1992). Cognitive and attitudinal impacts of university AIDS course: interdisciplinary education as a public health intervention. *American Journal of Public Health*; 82: 569-572.

21. Thomas, L (1988). AIDS: an unknown distance still to go. *Scientific American*; 259: 152.

CHAPTER NINE

QUENCHING THE FIRES OF HIV/AIDS IN AFRICA

Improved health owes less to advances on medical science than to changes in the external environment and to a favourable trend in the standard of living. We are healthier than our ancestors not because of what happens when we are ill, but because we do not get ill.—**World Health Organization (1957)**.

At the conclusion of Chapter Seven, it was stated that because of the devastating effect of HIV/AIDS on the continent of Africa, it was appropriate to say that Africa is burning. However, because of the uneven distribution of HIV/AIDS cases over the continent, the analogy was drawn that some countries were facing a towering inferno, whereas others were facing a forest fire, and still others were facing a simmering under-brush. With the fire analogy then, the approach to the control of the HIV/AIDS epidemic in Africa should be similar to that of fighting a fire. In other words, the same sense of urgency individuals and communities attach to fires which are burning out of control should be attached to the fires of HIV/AIDS in Africa.

Fire fighters all over the world know that it takes a specific plan to put out a fire, and the plan depends upon the type of fire and its intensity. In this regard, the approach to a forest fire would be different from that of a family residence or a large factory

213

because of the potential for chemical explosion in the latter. The final aim, however, is the ultimate quenching of the fire. In a forest fire, for example, the first step in putting out the fire may be the clearing the vegetation to create a clear path around the burning area, something fire fighters refer to as "constructing a firewall". This is done to prevent the fire from further spreading to adjacent areas, to stop the fire in its tracks, so to speak. Then water is poured on the fire to quench it. Often the creating of the fire wall and the actual quenching are done simultaneously with different groups of fire fighters.

In a forest fire, water is not the only tool used to quench it. Depending upon the size of the forest being burnt and intensity of the fire, many different tools, large and small, are employed. For example, bulldozers or machetes may be used to clear vegetation; axes or chain saws may be used to cut down trees; or bulldozers and pickaxes and shovels may be used to dig trenches around the fire, all in the process of creating the firewall. Sometimes sand or dirt is thrown on the fire in addition to or instead of water. And buckets, hoses, or even helicopters and airplanes may be used to douse the fire with water. In addition to size and intensity of the fire, what tools are employed depend upon what tools are available. For example, if there is no source of water available in the immediately vicinity of the fire, sand or dirt may be used to put out the fire.

In order to quench the fire of HIV/AIDS in Africa, there is the need to decide what type of fire it is. Also to be decided are the tools to be employed, taking into consideration the "intensity of the fire" and availability of "tools"... resources. The question of resources involves "helicopters, airplanes, bulldozers, buckets, axes, etc" as well as "trained fire fighters"; and it should employ "professional fire fighters" and "volunteer fire fighters".

I would liken the effect of HIV/AIDS on the continent of Africa to a wild forest that is burning out of control and covering a wide area. Like a real forest fire, there are areas of very high intensity, let's say "hot spots"; and there are areas that are not so hot. When fighting a forest fire, the whole fire, areas of higher intensity and of lower, are all completely quenched so as not to leave small fires that could simmer and become bigger ones later and spread. Like a real forest fire, a strategic plan needs to be developed, and the plan should be multifaceted. In other words, the plan should employ "bulldozer, machetes, axes, chain saws, pick axes, and shovels"; it should employ "helicopters, airplanes, hoses, and buckets"; and it should involve "professional and volunteer fire fighters".

With the above discussion, the practical "scientific" approach to HIV/AIDS in Africa, indeed in every part of the world, should be rather obvious. It should involve control and prevention; that is, putting out the fires that are already burning, and preventing the spread of the fire in terms of new infections. In other words, those living with HIV/AIDS should be treated, and those uninfected should be protected from the condition by "clearing vegetation or digging trenches to create a firewall" to protect them from infection. The ideal approach to fire fighting involves the creation of the firewall before quenching the fire itself. Thus, the HIV/AIDS epidemic should be contained through preventive measure before controlling it through therapeutic measures; or, at the very least, both therapeutic and preventive measures should be carried out simultaneously. But that has not been the case, as discussed in the last chapter.

As discussed in the last chapter, a lot of time has been wasted because of too much emphasis on drugs and vaccines. The problem in Africa is that the time wasted was due to both general inertia and a focus on the unavailability of drugs. Whereas a few countries focused on primary prevention and achieved demonstrable results, the rest either did nothing or spent a lot of time fighting for drugs that were not forthcoming. Then, in the case of South Africa, a lot of time was wasted on the debate over whether HIV caused AIDS, in addition to fighting for those drugs.

Obviously no more time should be wasted. The fires have to be quenched, the epidemic has to be controlled, with strategic planning. Recall that the goal of controlling an epidemic is twofold: (1) to improve the condition of those living with the disease, and (2) to use preventive measures to protect those without the disease from getting it. The overall approach should be that of prevention; that is, primary prevention to ensure that those not exposed to HIV remain free of exposure, secondary prevention to ensure that those already infected with HIV do not progress too soon to AIDS, and tertiary prevention to ensure that AIDS patients live as long and healthy a life as possible. I have suggested that the strategic plan should have four components: (1) treatment of HIV/AIDS, (2) counseling and testing, (3) research, and (4) education (Duh, 1991). The WHO declaration quoted above should serve as the backbone of the control effort.

As discussed in earlier chapters, the general health of an individual is an important determinant to the acquisition of HIV infection and progression to AIDS. Indeed, this attribute is important in the pathogenesis of most infectious and other diseases. Thus, as regards the WHO quotation above, changes in the external environment and a favourable standard of living vis-à-vis disease acquisition is very instructive. Many, perhaps most, Africans enjoy a relatively poor external environment and standard of living. Many of them are not much healthier than their ancestors, and it is they who are most often afflicted by *all kinds of diseases* including HIV/AIDS. Therefore, in order to succeed in controlling the HIV/AIDS epidemic in Africa, there needs to be a comprehensive approach.

The comprehensive approach should take into consideration the unique features of Africans infected and affected by HIV/AIDS. It should be based on both the biological and socio-economic reasons involving HIV/AIDS in Africa as discussed in chapters six and seven. The role of the subtypes of HIV found in Africa, other STIs, poverty, prostitution, polygamy, and traditional practices in the epidemic has to be considered. Then the comprehensive approach should be based on the four components of the strategic plan. I believe this approach can be effective in controlling the epidemic. But so far Africans with HIV/AIDS have been less involved in treatment, counseling and testing, research, and education. Why have Africans been less involved in the four components?

The issue with treatment involving HIV/AIDS has been almost exclusively discussed in terms of antiretroviral medications. There has been a lot of discussion in both the scientific and popular media about the lack of availability of these medications in Africa. With the exception of a few countries such as Senegal, Botswana and Uganda, the availability of these medications to most HIV/AIDS sufferers in African countries is very minimal at best. And the biggest obstacle to acquiring them is price (Flores, 2001). The actual cost of these drugs plus the cost of frequent blood tests and doctor visits attendant to the treatment with antiretroviral medications approaches US$20,000 a year. This is simply out of reach of most individuals and governments in Africa.

Many stakeholders in the HIV/AIDS arena have decried this "haves versus have-nots" phenomenon. Whereas most HIV/AIDS patients in developed countries are living longer and healthier lives because of these medicines, their counterparts in African countries are dying. So various stakeholders including governments, international organizations, and AIDS activists have declared this phenomenon as unacceptable. They have put pressure on the multinational pharmaceutical companies, who control these medicines, to make them available and affordable in African countries. Because of this pressure, the pharmaceutical companies made small, albeit significant, gestures.

Some of the companies offered selected drugs to selected countries free of charge for a period of time; and several of them offered to discuss substantial reductions in cost. When the offers were not widely embraced, they offered the drugs at about 10% the cost in developed countries, but these gestures were deemed inadequate by the various stakeholders. They wanted the drugs to be available everywhere at even lower prices then the 10% proposition. Furthermore, they wanted access to less expensive generic equivalents of these drugs. But the drug companies were not ready to give up their intellectual property rights. In this regard, Ghana and South Africa found themselves at loggerheads with the multinational pharmaceutical companies who controlled the antiretroviral medications.

The Indian generic pharmaceutical company, Cipla, had started selling a generic equivalent of Combivir (Lamivudine/ Zidovudine) in Ghana in the year 2000. Combivir was developed by the multinational pharmaceutical giant Glaxo-Wellcome, which held the patent to it. Not long afterwards, Glaxo-Wellcome promptly stopped Clipa from selling the generic version of Combivir in Ghana. The company sent a letter to both Clipa and the government of Ghana that Clipa's medicine was illegal because it violated Glaxo- Wellcome's patents (Global Health Council, 2001). The patent issue was more complicated in South Africa, and it received a lot of media attention. The issue ended up in court before it was finally resolved.

The government of South Africa had passed a law in 1997 that would allow South Africa to circumvent patent laws and import or manufacture less expensive generic medications in an emergency. Named the Medicines Control Act, the law was not put into force because of court challenges. The pharmaceutical companies argued that the law undermined their patents, and it was unconstitutional. They further argued that the patented drugs could be made available and affordable in South Africa with a combination of programmes.

In May 2000 several companies including Boehringer Ingelheim of Germany, Roche of Switzerland, Bristol-Myers

Squibb of the United States, and Glaxo-Wellcome of Britain offered to cut drug prices in developing countries. This offer was not taken up by the government of South Africa. Then in February 2001 Boehringer Ingelheim offered to supply South Africa with Viramune (Nevirapine) free of charge for five years. The free Viramune was to be used to prevent mother-to-child transmission of HIV in pregnant women. And Bristol-Myers Squibb offered a combination of its drugs Videx (Didanosine) and Zerit (Stavudine) for US$1 a day in South Africa. Both offers were not taken up (CNN/AP, 2001). Finally, a dramatic court proceeding took place in April 2001 in South Africa.

Thirty-nine multinational pharmaceutical companies and the Pharmaceutical Manufacturers' Association of South Africa had sued the government of South Africa to block the implementation of the Medicines Control Act (CNN/Reuters, 2001). For several days, lawyers on both sides argued their case in a packed courtroom in Pretoria. Hundreds of protestors displayed their dissatisfaction with the drug manufacturers by their presence inside the courtroom and outside. Their placards and chants accused the drug makers of putting profits ahead of human life. Several international organizations and prominent individuals including the former South African president, Nelson Mandela, added their voices to the chorus of protests. The companies issued various statements outside the courtroom setting to explain their stance as the proceedings went on. Then all of a sudden, the companies dropped their suit on April 19, 2001, bowing to the enormous pressure from so many sources.

In addition to discussions with individual countries, other fora took place at the international level for the discussion of price reduction by the drug companies. For example, the United Nations Secretary General, Kofi Annan, had discussions with six major drug companies on price reduction on April 5, 2001. The companies agreed to continue reducing prices for their antiretroviral medications to be affordable in poor countries. Mr. Annan could not divulge financial details of the agreement because of the companies' worry about being accused of antitrust violation (Reuters, 2001). Another forum took place in Norway the same month.

From April 8 to 11, 2001 a workshop was convened in Hosbjor, Norway, by the WHO, WTO (World Trade Organization), the Global Health Council, and the government of Norway. The purpose of the workshop was to discuss differential pricing of life-saving medications in poor countries. The idea behind differential pricing is that the pharmaceutical companies would sell drugs at different prices in different countries. By so doing, drugs would be sold at prices low enough for a particular country to afford while maintaining the regular prices in developed countries. Eighty experts from several groups including the pharmaceutical industry, multi lateral agencies, non-governmental organizations, and consumer groups attended the workshop. And after three days of deliberations, they concluded that the provision of drugs to poor countries was possible through differential pricing (Flores, 2001).

With the case against South Africa now settled, and the discussion at the UN and in Norway on reduced prices, African countries should be able to avail themselves of HIV/AIDS medications. Presumably, they could get the drugs in the form of less expensive generic equivalents or affordable brand name ones. In deed President Thabo Mbeki of South Africa was making arrangements for the importation of generic drugs before the case against his government was settled. He signed a series of agreements during a visit to Cuba in March 2001 with his Cuban counterpart, Fidel Castro, for the two countries to cooperate in producing generic drugs for HIV/AIDS. However, many experts believe that just making the drugs available and affordable is not enough.

Recall from earlier chapters that for drug therapy management to be effective, the particular drugs should be available, affordable, and *accessible*. There has to be the accessible health system infrastructure so that all or most people needing the drugs should get them. This fact was reiterated by the participants of the Norway workshop; and the then WHO Director-General Gro Harlem Brundtland added: "We have heard quite clearly that drug prices matter.... But little progress will be possible without a significant investment in building health systems" (Flores, 2001; p.4).

Accessibility also entails the availability of health professionals with the requisite experience with these drugs and the general management of HIV disease. These professionals should be able to identify and deal with drug side effects, compliance issues, and drug resistance. Another link in the accessibility equation is the uncontrolled nature of prescription drugs in many African countries. As stated in Chapter Four, all kinds of medicines can be obtained in most countries in Africa without prescription. Then they may be hoarded or shared with friends and relatives. Obviously this practice can accelerate the development of resistance to any drug; and it can really be bad news for powerful antiretroviral medications.

Dan Fountain has expressed his concern about the issue of uncontrolled prescription drugs based on his experience as a physician in Zaire (now the Democratic Republic of Congo) where prescription drugs could be obtained in pharmacy shops, on street corners, and open markets without a doctor's written prescription. In a powerful editorial, Dr. Fountain stated: "I believe that this issue must be dealt with before AIDS medicines are made generally available. We should require all nations to put into place adequate supervision of all pharmaceutical products. They should then be able to demonstrate adequate application of this supervision so that no prescription item should ever be found in a village market or unauthorized pharmacy." (Fountain, 2001; p.9).

Obviously, a lot of time has been spent on the issue of unavailability of antiretroviral medications in Africa. From the above discussion, it appears that more time would have to be spent putting plans in place before these drugs can be available on a wide-spread basis in Africa. Though the cost of antiretroviral medications has come down considerably to less than US$300 per month in many African countries, as of December 2005, only about 11% of the nearly five million people needing the medicines in sub-Saharan Africa were getting them (UNAIDS, 2006). Meanwhile many people are dying while others are suffering from HIV/AIDS, and still others are getting newly infected daily. But people with HIV/AIDS cannot and should not wait; they have to be treated, and the other components of the strategic plan should be implemented.

Like antiretroviral medications, counseling and testing activities have been rather limited in Africa. This situation has arisen largely because of the perception that counseling and testing programmes are of little value in the context of unavailability of drugs. The purpose of counseling and testing is to identify people with HIV infection at the asymptomatic stage and counsel those testing negative to take the necessary precautions to avoid infection. Then those testing positive are given treatment so as to delay the onset of AIDS for as long as possible. So it is not unreasonable to ask what the point of testing for HIV is if those testing positive cannot be offered treatment.

As regards research on HIV/AIDS in Africa, a lot of it has been by researchers from Western countries who go to some countries in Africa for short periods of time to conduct specific research. As stated in the last chapter, large-scale research similar to the U.S. AIDS Clinical Trials Group and the European Concorde Trials has not taken place in Africa. Some have suggested that the lack of large-scale research activities is a demonstration of a lack of interest in Africans with AIDS (DeCock et al, 1993). This is akin to the accusation of multinational pharmaceutical companies of putting profits ahead of human life by not making antiretroviral medications available in Africa. The exception to this phenomenon is in Kenya where African scientists have conducted research for international consumption.

Kenyan scientists conducted research on the use of Interferon to treat HIV disease. At the time Western scientists were experimenting with injectable Interferon as an adjunct to the treatment of HIV disease, the Kenyan scientists conducted studies on an oral form of Interferon called Kemron. Developed by American researchers and produced by a Japanese company, Kemron was used by scientists at the Kenya Medical Research Institute to treat AIDS patients. After one year of experimental use, the patients reported overall improvement in well-being, improvement in appetite and weight gain, and improvement in strength. Also the scientists observed alleviation of symptoms and increased CD4 count. The government of Kenya approved the general use of Kemron to treat AIDS in July 1990. But Kemron was not used in other countries purportedly because no other researchers could duplicate the result of the Kenyan researchers (Duh, 1991). Also in the last chapter is a discussion of vaccine research activity in Kenya. So in the desert of research activity in Africa on HIV/AIDS, Kenya has been an oasis of sorts.

What about the situation with education? It appears that of the four components of the strategic plan, education has been the one utilized the most in Africa. In this regard, Uganda, Kenya and Zimbabwe have achieved significant declines in adult prevalence due to behaviour change with respect to increase in condom use, decrease in multiple sexual partnerships, and delay in sexual debut by young people (UNAIDS, 2006). Yet prevention education has not been entrenched on a widespread basis and behaviour change has been rare. Thus, a lot of time has been wasted in Africa through inertia and unnecessary argument.

Meanwhile, Africa continues to burn with new HIV infections and deaths from AIDS. Without a doubt, there can be no more delays, no more time wasted. How do we save Africa from being burnt by HIV/AIDS? Where we go from here?

Where Do We Go From Here?

To answer this question, we need to consider where we have been and where we currently are. These two parameters have been discussed in this and other chapters. It is obvious that we have not been very far as regards the control of the HIV/AIDS epidemic in Africa. And we are at a critical point, a point where some communities face possible decimation, where the survival of the whole continent is threatened. This threat has to be arrested and arrested quickly by the strategic plan involving the four components.

Management of HIV disease.

It should be clear from previous discussions that the management of HIV/AIDS requires much more than just antiretroviral medications. The impact of the disease on patients is so profound that it requires a comprehensive approach, and the comprehensive approach should have prevention as its basis. The prevention approach is particularly relevant in Africa because of the unavailability of antiretroviral medications. Furthermore, because of the complications attendant to the antiretroviral medications, careful planning should be undertaken, and the appropriate infrastructure should be put in place, before making them the centre of treatment in Africa. How then should African

HIV/AIDS patients be treated? They should be treated as described in the last chapter with modifications for the special circumstances in Africa.

Recall that AIDS patients do not die directly from HIV; they die from opportunistic diseases as a result of the destruction of the immune system by HIV. Therefore, patients should ideally be identified early in the disease process and treatment instituted before they progress to AIDS. But treatment does not necessarily mean the use of antiretroviral medications. Treatment should focus on the use of other mechanisms to maximize the immune and general health status such as proper nutrition, exercise and adequate rest, stress management, and the provision of social services. Of particular importance is the prevention and treatment of endemic diseases which task the immune system such as STIs, malaria, TB, acute respiratory infections, and gastrointestinal diseases. Obviously, where they are available, antiretroviral medications should be utilized in conjunction with the other measures.

At the initial presentation, all patients diagnosed with HIV should be screened for TB by undergoing tuberculin skin testing. Those testing positive should be evaluated by chest x-ray and sputum test for active tuberculosis. If active TB is diagnosed, multi-drug treatment should be instituted, and those with just reactive skin test should receive prophylaxis. Similarly, they should be screened and treated for syphilis, chancroid, herpes, and other STIs. Close health care follow-up with regular visits to the doctor or clinic is paramount. There should be blood testing for CD4 count and other laboratory values at these visits. And when acute illnesses are diagnosed, they should be treated immediately. They should be vaccinated against meningitis, hepatitis A and B, tetanus, and measles (in susceptible individuals). All these are done to forestall the development of AIDS for as long as possible.

When the CD4 count reaches below 200 cells/mm, the patient is considered to have AIDS whether or not opportunistic infections are present. At this stage, the patients must be considered for antiretroviral medications if available and followed as described above for dealing with ARVs. Then the focus is on the management, that is, the prevention and treatment, of opportunistic infections. Doctor follow-ups should be more frequent, and the visits should be more structured and intense. All AIDS patients should be given PCP (*pneumocystis carinii pneumonia*) prophylaxis, though PCP may not be very common in some parts of Africa. Studies have shown that cryptosporidiosis, cryptococcal meningitis, herpes simplex virus infection, tuberculosis, and diarrhoeal diseases are the more common opportunistic infections in Africa, whereas American and European AIDS patients tend to have PCP and other pneumonias more often (Duh, 1991). They should also receive prophylaxis for candidiasis.

Until a true cure, that is, the elimination of HIV, can be achieved, the management of HIV/AIDS in Africa should be similar to that of other chronic diseases such as hypertension and diabetes, with the goal of living with (instead of dying from) the disease. Therefore, patients should be viewed *in toto* as far as treatment is concerned. Everything should be done to keep them as healthy and comfortable as possible in order to prevent the development of opportunistic infections. In this regard, nutritional status is very important because malnutrition is a major contributing factor to deaths from AIDS in Africa. Appetite enhancers such as Megesterol, Cyproheptadine, and Dronabinol should be offered to the patients. And nutritional supplements such as Ensure, Sustical, and Boost should be offered. These are balanced nutritional drinks that could be taken in addition to or instead of regular meals, particularly when appetite is not so good. They should also be offered other supplements such as multiple vitamins, iron, and folic acid on individual basis. Finally, they should stay away from sick people or situations where exposure to communicable diseases is likely.

Once opportunistic infections occur, they should be treated promptly and aggressively. The measures discussed in the last paragraph should be continued and intensified. With the opportunistic infections (and sometimes even before their onset), diarrhoea and nausea/vomiting are quite common among HIV/AIDS patients. Diarrhoea and vomiting are very dangerous in that they interfere with the absorption of medicines, nutrients, and supplements; and they can cause death because of dehydration. They must be prevented and treated comprehensively with medications and fluids as needed.

A final component to the chronic management of HIV/AIDS is psychological counseling. The chronic, debilitating, and devastating nature of HIV/AIDS makes its victims prone to psychological problems. Lost relationships, lost jobs, and lost housing are quite common among these patients; and these losses often lead to a lot of stress for the patients. This is even more of a problem in Africa where many people believe that HIV/AIDS is the act of witchcraft or God.

The stigmatisation and shame attached to the disease, along with the losses listed above, often cause profound psychological stress. This in turn adversely affects the immune system, general health status, and even how treatment may work. It is also possible that the burden of the psychological stress may cause some HIV/AIDS patients to act irresponsibly. For example, the gentleman quoted in Chapter Seven as saying that he did not ask for it (HIV infection), so he would spread it around might have said that out of frustration because of the psychological burden of the disease. Obviously, dealing with this aspect of the disease is of paramount importance.

Counseling and Testing.

As stated earlier, some may question the need for testing someone for HIV infection if the person cannot be offered antiretroviral treatment. But as discussed above, one does not need antiretroviral medications in order to treat HIV/AIDS. Indeed, there is a more fundamental reason than treatment to test someone for HIV—counselling. The purpose of the counseling is to effect primary and secondary prevention. For primary prevention, those testing positive would be counseled on measures to take so as not to expose others to the virus; and for secondary prevention, these people would receive counseling on measures to keep themselves healthy, and be provided prophylaxis and other treatment to prevent progression to AIDS. Again, in countries where antiretroviral medications are available and the appropriate health system infrastructure exists, they should be given the ARVs to complement other treatment modalities in a comprehensive approach. Then those testing negative would be counseled on precautions to take to avoid exposure.

The most widely available tests for HIV infection are the ELISA and the Western Blot tests to detect antibodies to HIV. When the tests were licensed in 1985, it was recommended that they be done with pre-test and post-test counseling, and that recommendation has been carried through until now. In some situations, it may be inconvenient or difficult to conduct both pre-test and post-test counseling, but the counseling is very important. People undergoing the testing should fully understand what the test is supposed to detect. For example, I have had patients ask me for an AIDS test. The implication of this request is that if the test is positive, then the person has AIDS. Obviously, this is wrong; the ELISA and Western blot blood tests are to detect antibodies to HIV, *the virus that causes AIDS*. People should also clearly understand what negative and positive antibody test results mean.

As discussed in Chapter Three, there could be a "lag" time of about six months from HIV infection to the presence of antibodies in the blood stream. Therefore, people testing negative for HIV antibodies may actually be infected. Thus, it is imperative that those testing negative fully understand the lag time phenomenon and take appropriate precautions. Even if the result is a true reflection of a negative test, the person should not use it as a licence for reckless behaviour, and the provider should take the opportunity to counsel about how to avoid the contraction of HIV and other STIs. They should be screened and treated for STIs since these diseases potent increased risk for contracting HIV infection.

When the test is positive, counseling should be provided on proper nutrition, stress management, proper exercise and rest, and avoidance of STIs and other cofactor diseases. People with positive results should quickly be placed into some health care system if they do not already have a doctor. In some situations, it may be necessary to refer to providers who are more knowledgeable about and comfortable with treating HIV/AIDS. Then they should be followed regularly for check-ups and treatment of all diseases likely to effect progression to AIDS. They should also be tested immediately and regularly thereafter for CD4 count and other blood values as discussed in the last section. The need for all these follow-up activities should be fully explained during the post-test counseling session.

Another important issue to be discussed during the post-test counseling session is partner notification. This is particularly important in situations where there may be more than one partner. The person testing positive should be encouraged to inform all partners about the result and implore them to get tested *and* take appropriate precautions. In addition, the provider should obtain names, addresses, and telephone numbers, when available, for all partners during the post-test counseling session. The provider should then seek the client's permission to inform the partners. If the provider is to inform the partners, the client should be assured that their name would not be used. They should also be assured of complete confidentiality as regards employers and family members; disclosure of the test results to other people should be left completely up to the clients.

In consideration of the purpose of testing and counseling, ideally everyone in the population should be tested for maximum benefit for the control of the epidemic. Obviously, this is not practical, and selective testing has been recommended. In this regard, the term *voluntary counselling and testing* (VCT) has been in vogue; that is, individuals would voluntarily ask to be tested. But as part of a major effort to control the epidemic that is threatening a whole continent, depending on people to volunteer for testing seems rather inadequate. In Western countries, some have advocated testing all people in high-risk groups such as homosexuals, drug users, and prostitutes. The problem with this approach is that those outside these groups might not go for testing by believing that they cannot get HIV.

An alternative selective approach is what I term *focused testing*; that is, focusing on selected groups of people in selected areas. For example, testing may be offered to everyone attending STI clinics, hospital inpatients, pregnant women attending antenatal clinic, and some groups of young people such as university students. Another approach to focused testing is visiting workers at their place of employment to discuss testing. In this regard, industries and other firms or companies, both private and governmental, with a large number of young workers may be targeted. People belonging to mobile populations such long distance drivers, iterant traders, mine workers and port workers may be targeted. In addition, prostitutes or commercial sex workers tend to have particularly high prevalence rates of HIV infection, and they should be visited for testing purposes. But the most important group to be targeted for testing in Africa should be pregnant women.

If a major purpose of testing for HIV infection is to be able to offer antiretroviral medications to those testing positive, then pregnant women are prime candidates for testing and counseling. Antiretroviral medications for general use to treat HIV/AIDS have been largely nonexistent in Africa mainly because of the cost. And because the problems enumerated earlier regarding these medicines, they are not likely to be available on large scale there soon. But taking one pill for very short periods of time has been shown to dramatically reduce mother-to-child or vertical transmission of HIV. Since 1994, the use of AZT and more recently that of Nevirapine in infected women during pregnancy and delivery, and giving them to their newborns, have been shown to protect as many as 95% of the children from vertical transmission. Because of this, it has been popular, at least in Western countries, to test pregnant women (Kass, 2000). Also, pregnant women testing positive would be counseled on breast-feeding, when appropriate, since breast-feeding is a significant mode of HIV transmission from mother to child.

Testing pregnant women has followed the same general guidelines for testing and counseling; that is, it has been voluntary and been accompanied by pre- and post-test counseling. Because of the voluntary nature, the test has often been offered to women who are perceived by providers to be at risk. But considering the potential benefit of the test, the United States Congress mandated the Institute of Medicine (IOM) in 1996 to come up with recommendations for testing to reach more pregnant women. An IOM committee recommended that HIV testing be incorporated into the panel of blood routinely drawn during pregnancy. This process would eliminate the pre-test counseling part of HIV testing. However, the women should be informed that the test is going to be done, and they might choose to refuse the test. The recommendations were adopted by the CDC for its new guidelines for pregnant women (Kass, 2000).

While the goal of the guidelines is to reach more people, they pose a potential ethical problem in that some providers may do the test without informing the women or may not give post-test counseling. Some women who find out after the fact that they have tested positive may suffer domestic abuse and stigmatisation (Kass, 2000). Nancy Kass has expressed her dilemma about the situation this way: "As an ethicist, to endorse a policy that may compromise informed consent for HIV testing with pregnant women is painful. *At the same time, it is more painful to watch HIV-infected babies be born to women who wanted to be tested and...never were offered HIV testing in their pregnancies.* (Kass, 2000; p. 1027) (Italics added).

I agree completely with Dr. Kass's statement, particularly the highlighted part. It is indeed painful to watch HIV-infected babies. It is bad enough to be a healthy orphan to AIDS parents, but to be born with HIV infection and lose a mother to AIDS is doubly painful. The case of Nkosi Johnson, the courageous AIDS orphan from South Africa, is an example of how bad things could be for AIDS orphans to be born HIV-infected. He was lucky to have had a caring adoptive mother who could provide him love

235

and other material means. Yet he suffered discrimination and humiliation; he was even prevented temporarily from attending school with other children. But for the support of his mother, well wishers, and his own courage and will to live, Nkosi would not have survived for as long as he did, dying at the age of 12. If a well-placed child like Nkosi Johnson could suffer that much from the double whammy of an AIDS orphan and AIDS victim, how does society deal with poor children without Nkosi's relative fortune in the same double whammy situation.

I believe the IOM recommendations should be adopted in all African countries and all pregnant women be tested for HIV infection. We should not worry too much about ethics at this critical juncture when it comes to the well being of unborn children vis-à-vis HIV infection. Important as ethics is, it is even more important that we control a terrible epidemic and save lives. Under normal circumstances, informed consent and pre-test counseling should precede HIV testing; but the HIV/AIDS situation in Africa is not "normal", and it requires aggressive and courageous action. After all, unusual situations call for unusual action, so let us do what is possible to curb or possibly eliminate one of the means of HIV transmission. This will help in the overall control of the HIV/AIDS epidemic in Africa by reducing the number of new cases.

Research.

Research is very important in the control of any epidemic, and it is even more necessary for the HIV/AIDS epidemic, particularly in Africa where research activity has not been very prominent. In addition to research on medications and vaccines, other epidemiological research should be ongoing as part of a comprehensive approach to the control of the epidemic. Of particular importance are prevalence studies. Data in many countries are obtained from the pools of individuals who voluntarily seek testing. Another source of data on HIV prevalence is sentinel studies of antenatal clinic attendants. These sources may not be representative of the population.

People seeking voluntary testing may be involved in behaviours that place them at a higher risk for HIV infection, and results here may not be representative of the community. On the other hand, some people may not consider themselves at risk and would not seek voluntary testing. Similarly, antenatal clinic attendees may have a different risk profile from the general population in that they are all women and may be of a lower social grouping since such studies are usually conducted at public clinics.

Special sero-prevalence studies, utilizing probability sampling techniques of different communities, would reach more people, and the results would more accurately reflect the HIV/AIDS problem in a community or country. Demographic and health surveys conducted periodically by the government could be utilized for this purpose. Academic institutions, non-governmental organizations (NGOs), and large companies may also conduct general sero-prevalence studies. Results of the studies will help in developing comprehensive plans for dealing with the epidemic, particularly with regard to education and treatment programmes.

In addition to the groups listed in the last section, all newborns, clients attending family planning clinics, TB patients, and selected students in particular catchment areas may be tested. In this situation, the participants would be informed that blood was being drawn for research purposes but would undergo pre- and post-test counseling. They should be assured of complete confidentiality and anonymity that their names would not appear in any published documents; only demographic data such as race, age, gender, and place of residence would be used. There should be laws or other provisions to deal with those who divulge testing results to people other than those being tested. Obviously, people testing positive should receive further counseling and referral to the nearest providers for disease management as discussed in the last section.

A concomitant of prevalence studies are surveillance studies. The purpose of surveillance is to provide information to effect actions. It involves the collection, collation, and analysis of data for prompt dissemination to those who need to know (Thacker et al, 1983). There should be surveillance workers who would be in direct contact with doctors, hospitals, clinics, and laboratories to collect up-to-date data on HIV infection and AIDS diagnosis in communities. They should also collect data on who are receiving treatment and the type of treatment being received. Then, there should be information on those not receiving treatment and why they are not receiving it (Duh, 1991). Surveillance activities would provide valuable information to local and national governments, academic and other health professionals, NGOs, and other policy makers in the HIV/AIDS arena for setting priorities and managing control programs.

A final research program should be attitudinal studies or behaviour surveillance. For example, in a study conducted by the

Ghana National AIDS Control Program, more than 90% of people surveyed stated they were aware of HIV/AIDS, but nearly 80% believed they personally or their families were not at risk for the condition (unpublished data). There should be studies to find out the reasons for such apparent inconsistency. There should be studies on people's attitudes regarding polygamy, prostitution, and traditional practices as they relate to the acquisition of HIV infection. There should be studies on the very serious issue of female circumcision, especially why some young females are for the procedure. Specifically, it should be found out if and how people want to change their attitude and behaviour regarding some of these practices. There should be studies on people's attitudes and behaviour about multiple sexual partnerships, abstinence from sex, and condom use. There should also be studies on the efficacy and safety of traditional medicines for HIV/AIDS and people's attitudes toward their use.

The research activities discussed above, in addition to others, are important in the control of the epidemic. Not only would the information help in the development of policy and budget allocation, the studies would provide an opportunity for education. Be it a prevalence study, surveillance study, or attitudinal study, the settings usually involve a captive audience, and the participants could be given individual counseling. They could also be educated to become educators (peer educators) for their families, friends, schoolmates, co-workers, and local communities.

Education.

Without a doubt, education is the most important component of the comprehensive program to control the HIV/AIDS epidemic in Africa. Education is indispensable to any prevention approach. Thus, whether we are dealing with treatment (or even a cure), testing and counseling, or research, education is key to success. It is even more important when there is no cure, and antiretroviral medications for treatment are not available. Modification of population and individual characteristics is the best or only way to control the epidemic, regardless of the level of prevention at which we are operating.

Education on HIV/AIDS should have two purposes: (1) to alleviate unfounded fears and clarify misconceptions about the disease, and (2) to arm people with tools to prevent HIV infection. Both purposes require the dissemination of accurate, up-to-date, and understandable information about the virus, HIV, and the disease, AIDS. To be effective, educational messages must be credible, consistent, persuasive, and often repeated (Duh, 1991).

The backbone of HIV/AIDS education should be the understanding of HIV disease at the basic biological level. People should be made to understand that HIV infection is caused by a virus or germ, just as a virus or germ causes measles or malaria. It is not caused by punishment from God or by evil spirits and witchcraft. Therefore, HIV/AIDS victims should be treated with the same care and compassion as measles and malaria victims. The biology of HIV infection should be explained in terms of simple virology, immunology, transmission, pathogenesis, and treatment. Then prevention should be discussed in relation to behaviours that effect transmission and how to avoid or modify those behaviours. Particular attention should be paid to individual responsibility regardless of the audience. Obviously, the level of technical and frank sexual language used would depend upon the audience and the setting.

Like the other components of the strategic plan, education should be comprehensive and community based. It should take place at a variety of settings including schools, homes, workplace, churches, hospitals, and clinics. "HIV/AIDS libraries" may be set up at these places, local libraries, and community centres. Printed, audio, and video material in appropriate local languages would be available at the "libraries" to disseminate understandable and useful information on HIV/AIDS. Community fora and symposia should be organized frequently during which experts or people quite well versed on the topic, preferably from the community, are invited to discuss various aspects of the HIV/AIDS issue. Every member of the society should be educated regardless of one's potential risk of actually contracting the virus.

The ultimate aim of the educational programs is to effect lasting behavioural and attitudinal change. Therefore, with the information on biology of HIV/AIDS, people should be taught to modify beliefs and behaviours that put them and others at risk of contracting HIV. For example, there should be a revolutionary change in the belief that young people must have sex, that multiple sexual partnerships is okay or even necessary, that females should make their vagina dry for men's sexual pleasure, that female circumcision must be a right of passage.

The issue of sex and sexuality is very important in the education process, particularly as it relates to the youth. Young people should be taught very early about sex and sexuality in biological terms with emphasis on debunking myths perpetuated by peers. They should be taught that it is okay to wait until marriage to indulge sex. The ABC approach, which stands for **A**bstinence, **B**e faithful to your partner, **C**ondom use, should be utilized in the education on sex and sexuality.

The approach calls for abstaining from sex since that is the only absolutely sure way of avoiding contracting HIV infection. Therefore, abstinence must be stressed to the youth, and ways to help them abstain should be explored. If (and only if) one cannot abstain from sex, then one must have only one partner and ensure that that partner is not having sex with anyone else. And if (and only if) one cannot abstain or remain faithful to a partner, then condom use is the next best option.

It should be understood that condom use is the only available tool to reduce one's chance for the sexual transmission of HIV. So there should not be too much discussion on whether or not it is 100% effective, and whether or not it promotes promiscuity. There are numerous studies that demonstrate that condom promotion does not lead to increased sexual activity. Then both male and female condoms must be made available, affordable, and accessible.

Of paramount importance is the teaching of the proper and consistent use of condoms; then the enabling environment must be created so that people would feel free to acquire and use them. For example, for some males, to use condoms and for some females, to ask their partners to use them means that there is something wrong with them or they are not being faithful to their partner. They must be disabused of those beliefs. Also, some young people want to use condoms but they are shy or embarrassed to ask for them at a pharmacy. They should be taught to get rid of such feelings; and condoms should be made available in ways that people could get to without having to ask. Furthermore, for some people, no matter how low the prices of condoms are, they might not be able to afford them. Free condoms should be made available as much as possible.

Perhaps the biggest roadblock on the path of controlling the HIV/AIDS epidemic is the problem of stigmatisation and discrimination. From the very beginning of the epidemic, people with the condition have suffered stigmatisation and discrimination. Because of the stigma attached to the disease, people with the condition have suffered all kinds of discrimination. Even worse is that the discrimination often touches both the people infected and those affected by the condition; that is, relatives and friends of HIV/AIDS patients may suffer similar discrimination to that of patients themselves.

People with HIV/AIDS may be denied housing; may be divorced from marriage by uninfected spouses; may be denied health care; may be abandoned by family and friends; or may be dismissed from school. There are even stories of people actually boycotting funerals of AIDS victims! In short, many people living with HIV/AIDS are being denied their basic human rights.

Why are HIV/AIDS victims so often stigmatized and discriminated against? This probably stems from the fact that the epidemic started from the homosexual and drug use communities. Homosexuality and illicit drug use have always been viewed by many people as sinful or immoral. Therefore, people did not want to be associated with a disease affecting "sinners". Then when the condition started surfacing in other communities, the stigma continued because of the relationship between the condition and sexual intercourse. Somehow, many people view sexually transmitted disease as shameful or even sinful. Thus, stigmatisation and discrimination have accompanied the evolution of the epidemic until now. My personal observation has led me to conclude that the perpetuation of HIV/AIDS stigmatisation and discrimination is based on the following:

- The view that victims deserve their fate because they did something wrong to get the disease
- The view that there is no cure for the disease....they are going to die, anyway (so let them die)
- Unfounded fears about HIV/AIDS
- Lack of adequate knowledge about the disease process

HIV/AIDS sufferers deserve their fate because of immoral acts or doing something wrong.

To say that people with HIV/AIDS deserve their fate is a display of ignorance and prejudice. First of all, not everyone who has HIV did something "wrong". What did the baby do wrong when she was infected in the womb or during birth or from breast-feeding? What did the married woman do wrong when she remained faithful to her husband and the husband, let's say a long distance truck driver, contracted HIV somewhere and gave it to her? What did the farmer do wrong when he was given HIV-infected blood transfusion during surgery for a hernia repair?

On the other hand, if we say that the long distance driver who got HIV because he was not faithful to his wife should be stigmatized or denied care, then we should do the same for almost everyone who is ill because almost every illness results from what we do or do not do to ourselves. Do we deny medical care to people who smoke cigarettes and get pneumonia or lung cancer? Do we deny care to people who drink alcohol in excess and get liver disease? Do we deny care to people who eat too much fatty food and do not exercise and get heart disease? Do we deny care to people who drink and drive and get seriously injured in motor accidents? Even something like malaria that results from mosquito bite results from our own negligence—for creating or allowing conditions that breed mosquitoes or not sleeping under bed nets. Yes; almost every human illness results from our "doing something wrong."

HIV/AIDS sufferers should be left to die because there is no cure for it.

Do we deny people care and stigmatize them when other diseases they have are not curable? If we did that, then we would let almost every sick person die because almost every illness is incurable. There is no cure for hypertension, asthma, diabetes, most cancers, arthritis, stroke, heart disease, emphysema, etc. People with such diseases are given treatment, often different kinds of medication, to control the diseases so that the patients can have relatively normal lives. These people will die if the medication is stopped or is not taken properly. In other words, people with these chronic diseases would die without effective treatment, just as people with AIDS would die without effective treatment. We are talking about treatment, not cure. Therefore, we should treat people with HIV/AIDS with the same care and compassion as we treat those with other chronic incurable but treatable diseases.

Unfounded fears about the disease.

HIV/AIDS is perhaps the most feared disease in the world. People are so afraid of the disease that they behave irrationally. Some people would rather commit suicide than to get AIDS. Because of this profound fear, some people would go to any extent to avoid HIV/AIDS patients. This has led to all kinds of discrimination, including being denied housing and health care, being divorced from marriages, being abandoned by family and friends, and even having their funerals boycotted. Despite the fact that it has been trumpeted since the onset of the epidemic that one cannot get AIDS by touching, shaking hands, eating and talking with people with HIV/AIDS, people continue to harbour fears about the disease; and these kinds of discrimination stem from those fears. And I believe these fears are a result of lack of adequate knowledge about the disease process.

Lack of knowledge about the disease process

The approach to education about HIV/AIDS in many countries often involves the stating of facts; that is, people are given facts instead of understandable information. For example, we say that one cannot get AIDS by touching an AIDS patient, but we do not explain why not. This approach leads to superficial and shallow perception of the problem and does not lead to behavior and attitudinal change. People need to be given understandable

246

information, and people need to take the time to absorb, digest and assimilate such information. Once they have a more complete understanding of the disease process, they are less likely to have unfounded fears about touching, shaking hands, eating and talking with people with HIV/AIDS. Thus, just as education is paramount to the control of the HIV/AIDS epidemic in general, it is key to the reduction of stigmatization and discrimination attached to the epidemic.

The discussion above on the four components is based on a theoretical framework. To state, for example, that AIDS patients should be offered appetite enhancers and nutritional supplements or prophylactic medications, pre-supposes that those items are available to be offered and there are providers to offer them. Also, to state that HIV/AIDS patients should have regular doctor visits for blood tests and treatment or be provided with psychological counseling, pre-supposes that such personnel and facilities are available. Admittedly, the availability, affordability, and accessibility problems attendant to antiretroviral medications also exist for the other management issues. Therefore, the problem of availability, affordability, and accessibility should be handled in conjunction with the comprehensive program.

Many experts agree that effective health care system infrastructure should be put in place before antiretroviral medications should be provided in African countries on a large scale basis. I have argued that we cannot and should not wait, but we should employ the other tools discussed above to manage HIV/AIDS patients and offer primary prevention programs to those not infected to remain uninfected. Though these other management options require an effective health care system infrastructure, I believe that existing systems can handle them while steps are being taken to improve the whole system. In most cases, the services discussed above can be provided in the current system, with some modification and adjustment.

Finally, there should be an attempt to obtain some of the medications and supplies for the prevention and treatment of opportunistic diseases. Some of the medicines such as Fluconazole, Megesterol, and Dronabinol are very expensive, costing more than $100 for a month's supply in the United States. Also the food supplements such as Ensure and Boost are quite expensive. For example, Ensure is recommended to be taken three cans a day, and the three cans cost more than $4. That means one needs 90 cans a month, and that amounts to more than $120. Obviously, these costs are well beyond the means of most individuals and even governments in Africa. Though these medicines and supplements are expensive, they are not as expensive as the antiretroviral medications. And in some ways they may be more valuable to the patient than the antiretroviral medications.

So while exploring sources of financial and in kind support to deal with the HIV/AIDS epidemic, individual African governments should target the pharmaceutical companies that produce these drugs and supplies. In the same manner that some of the companies have agreed to reduce the prices of antiretroviral medications or give them out free of charge, they would agree to do the same for the management of opportunistic diseases.

I have been talking about the need to focus on the management of opportunistic disease in lieu of or in addition to the treatment of HIV with antiretroviral medication in my speeches for some time. In these speeches, I make mention of the fact that African governments and AIDS activists should target drug companies for medications and supplies for opportunistic diseases at substantial reductions or free. So I was delighted to hear of the announcement by the pharmaceutical giant, Pfizer, in June 2001 that it would supply the anti-fungal medication, Difflucan (Fluconazole), free of charge to people who needed it in Africa. I believe other companies would follow Pfizer's example if they were made aware of the need for their particular products.

REFERENCES

1. American Public Health Association (1996). UNAIDS offers global approach to epidemic. *The Nations Health, August* 1996; p.1, 18.
2. CNN/AP. S. Africa spurned AIDS drug offer. *Daily Graphic*, April 3, 2001; p. 5.
3. CNN/Reuters. Mandela slams drug makers, chides South African gov't. *Daily Graphic*, April 17 2001; p. 5.
4. DeCock, K.M. (1993). Clinical research, prophylaxis, therapy, and care of HIV disease. *American Journal of Public Health Assoc*; 83: 1385 - 1389.
5. Duh, S. V. (1991). *Blacks and AIDS: Causes and Origins*, Newbury Park: Sage Publications.
6. Flores, T. (2001). Drug summit: price is important. *Global HealthLink*; 109: 4.
7. Fountain, D. (2001). Problems with affordable AIDS medicine. *AIDSLinks*: 67: 8.
8. Global Health Council (2001). Glaxo enters fight in Ghana on AIDS drugs. *AIDSLinks*; 66:16.
9. Integrated Regional Information Networks. (2001). Cuba poised to enter generic AIDS drug market. *AIDSLinks*; 67: 7.

10. Kass, N. (2000). A change in approach to prenatal HIV screening. *American Public Health Assoc*; 90: 1026-1027.

11. Reuters. Major firms promise cheaper AIDS drugs. *Daily Graphic*; April 7, 2001.

12. Thacker, S.B. et al (1983). The surveillance of infectious diseases. *Journal American Medical Assoc.* 249: 1181-1186.

13. UNAIDS (2006). AIDS epidemic update: December 2005—sub-Saharan Africa

CHAPTER TEN

EDUCATING THE PUBLIC ON HIV/AIDS: WHOSE JOB IS IT?

The AIDS epidemic, perhaps understandably, was greeted with an emotional response when it first arrived on the scene in 1981. To control the epidemic, it became necessary to educate the public quickly. Indeed, before the causative agent for AIDS and drugs were discovered, education was the only tool for the control process. In the process of educating the public, facts, instead of understandable information, have been thrown at the public, and the public has often reacted to the facts emotionally. Therefore, after hearing about AIDS almost incessantly for more than 20 years, many people still demonstrate ignorance about it.

If the purpose of AIDS education is to effect attitudinal and behaviour change, then facts alone may not be enough to change minds. Some people need more convincing before they would change what may amount to lifelong beliefs and behaviours. It may not be enough, for example, to just say that one cannot get HIV infection by shaking hands with an HIV/AIDS patient or from a mosquito bite. That statement alone may not help remove the fear of shaking hands with AIDS patients or the belief that HIV can be transmitted through mosquito bites.

Similarly, it is not enough to just tell someone not to have sex with multiple partners or to use condom for sex. People need to know exactly why and, more importantly, how they should accomplish those things. For example, the discussion of the consistent and proper use of condoms is paramount in any educational effort to promote the widespread use of condoms. On the other hand, it appears that even those who accept the facts about HIV/AIDS may not necessarily know what exactly the facts mean.

In my speeches, especially when I am speaking to doctors and other health care personnel, I often state that they need to give understandable information instead of just facts when they talk to their clients about HIV/AIDS. For example, if they just tell someone that HIV is not transmitted through handshake, they have given a fact; if they explain why it is not transmitted that way, they have given understandable information. Then I pause and ask, "Can someone get AIDS by shaking hands with an AIDS patient?" Many people in the audience would shake their heads no. Then I would ask, "Why not?" And I often hear or see nothing. Those health professionals know and accept the fact that HIV is not transmitted through handshake but are not readily able to give the reasoning behind that statement. They might not have been properly informed and are unlikely to adequately inform their clients. Yes; education on HIV/AIDS is difficult and complex, but it must be done and done properly because it is indispensable to the control of the epidemic.

It has been emphasized from the beginning of the epidemic that education is the key to its control. So whose job is it to educate the public about HIV/AIDS? Studies have shown that most lay people get their information on HIV/AIDS from the popular media—radio, television, newspapers, and magazines. Other sources have been the schools, doctors and other health care professionals, families, churches, places of employment, and pamphlets/brochures. In addition, there are community-based organizations that offer structured HIV/AIDS education. How good are these "educators"? The answer appears to be not very good if one judges how good they are by the impact education has had on the epidemic. After more than 20 years of hearing about the disease, people all over the world still harbour unfounded fears, and people still indulge in behaviours and activities that place them at risk for acquiring HIV. Worse is that in some cases, some of the risky behaviours are on the increase.

Why do people continue to indulge in health-damaging or life threatening behaviour? Some researchers suggest that the problem may lie with entrenched human behaviour, not the inadequacy of HIV/AIDS education. For example, Jean Kalonoski, who was the director of HIV services for Planned Parenthood Association of New York in the United States, has stated: "I don't think we can blame the messengers or the way they have presented the message. We have to explore why people are not accepting what they are being told." (American Health Consultants, 1993: p. 88). The second part of Ms. Kalonoski's statement is instructive. We need to explore more the reasons behind human behaviour, why people indulge in self-destructive behaviour. For example, why do people continue to smoke cigarettes, eat excessive amounts of fat-laden food, drive while drunk...when the dangers involved are well known? And why do people continue to share needles or have unprotected sex with multiple partners without condoms when the dangers involved are known?

Dr. Harvey Finegold of Harvard University in the United States has suggested that sexual behaviour, for example, is biologically based and socially sanctioned. That makes it difficult to change (Finegold, 1988). Dr. Thomas Morris of Notre Dame University in the United States has discussed destructive behaviour on the basis of three philosophical viewpoints—ignorance, indifference, and inertia. On the basis of ignorance, people might not know that their behaviour is harmful, or if they have an idea, they may not know exactly what the problem may be. Indifference involves not being concerned about something, knowing that it is harmful. But Morris adds that this is a feigned indifference—the individual is not totally without concern but may be confused. Inertia is simply the power of habit; that is, people get stuck in a rut and are unable to get out of it (Morris, 1992).

An example of Morris's indifference principle is how I saw a young man react to the use of condoms on television. An American TV reporter was discussing the AIDS epidemic and the role of condom use in controlling it. He made a comment about the fact that most sexually active people did not use it, and he interviewed people who happened to come by where he was. One young man responded to the reporter's inquiry by saying that he did not like condoms and would never use them. He added: "I'd rather die than use a rubber." Obviously, this is a feigned indifference. Perhaps somewhere in the back of his mind, this young man had told himself that he would take his chances and have sex without condoms; hopefully he would not contract HIV in the process. However, if he knew that having sex without a condom would definitely kill him, he might not make such a statement. Another example is a story told to me by a university student in Ghana. He was giving away brochures around campus on responsible sexual behaviour when a male lecturer told him that when he met a beautiful girl, he cared nothing about AIDS or other STIs. Again, this lecturer might simply be playing Russian roulette with sex.

So what do we do about human behaviour in order to effect necessary changes? We cannot do nothing just because what people do is biologically based or we all do things based on inertia. I believe we should divide Morris's principles into two broad categories—ignorance, and indifference/inertia. Then we should explore the whys and hows of those principles as they relate to people's behaviour regarding HIV/AIDS. Exploration, of course, means research; and research should be conducted on human behaviour as relates to HIV/AIDS. Once research findings give an indication of why people do those certain things, then necessary steps should be taken to address those issues to effect the necessary behaviour change.

As important as or more important than research is the application of programs to teach people about HIV/AIDS in order to effect the necessary behaviour change. Whose job is it to do the teaching? The U.S. Public Health Service, UNAIDS, and others have advocated a multi-centric approach to the teaching. They have advocated the involvement of health professionals, schools (from elementary through university), churches, the media, community-based organizations, and families. All the experts agree that the most effective educational programs are community based.

Since the aim of HIV/AIDS education is to alleviate unfounded fears and to effect behaviour change to prevent the spread of HIV infection, the "teachers" enumerated above may play different roles. For example, the churches' and families' role may mainly be the teaching of abstinence from sex, illicit drug use, and alcohol use. Studies have shown that young people may be more responsive to their parents regarding sexual behaviour (Tucker, 1991). Health professionals, the schools, and the media are better positioned to teach the biology of HIV disease to alleviate fears and effect behaviour modification. And, of course, the best results are achieved when community-based programs draw on the strengths of all educators.

It is imperative that those who teach the biology of HIV/AIDS are themselves well-educated so they do not give just facts, or worse, misleading and false information. For example, media reports often state that someone has AIDS when the person has only HIV infection. It is important to distinguish between HIV infection and AIDS. Printed material should also be accurate in presenting HIV/AIDS information. For example, a sales representative of a commercial laboratory brought some brochures on HIV antibody testing to my office some time ago when I was working in the United States. The brochure entitled, *Health*

Facts: AIDS and Testing for HIV Antibodies was to be given to patients who might need HIV antibody testing. It contained this confusing statement: "AIDS is a serious condition *that weakens the body's immune system leaving it unable to fight off illnesses* (italics added). Obviously, weakened immune system is not caused by AIDS; it is caused by HIV, and AIDS *results from the weakened immune system.* Another statement in the brochure was outright wrong: "The HIV antibody test is *the only way* you can tell if you are infected" (italics added). HIV antibody test is not the only test for HIV infection; it is the most commonly used test because it is the easiest and cheapest test. Other tests such as *polymerase chain reaction* (PCR) or p24 antigen tests are more complicated and expensive, and thus not used for routine screening.

The problem of confusing HIV infection with AIDS has serious implications. People with just HIV infection may have no symptoms whatsoever and can perform usual activities including holding down a job. When they have AIDS, they are usually unable to work. Employers may believe falsely that their HIV-infected workers should be terminated if told the workers involved have AIDS. Also, the stigma attached to AIDS could lead to all kinds of discriminatory attitude towards AIDS patients. Some workers may not want to work next to an AIDS patient but may not mind being close to an HIV-infected person with no symptoms. Therefore, it is necessary to state that a person has just HIV infection, and it is even better to add that he or she does not have AIDS yet and is capable of functioning normally.

The irony about working next to an AIDS patient is that the healthy worker may pose a threat to the AIDS patient and not vice versa because the healthy worker may harbour an infectious condition which ordinarily does not bother him or her because of intact immune system. When such a condition is transmitted to the AIDS patient either through the air or by touching, it could threaten the life of the AIDS patient.

Media personnel are not the only educators who may have less than desirable knowledge about HIV/AIDS. Some doctors and other health care professionals may not have adequate knowledge on HIV/AIDS. I conducted a study in 1988 on AIDS knowledge on audiences of my oral presentations. Over a period of several months, I had members of the audience fill out a questionnaire prior to my speaking to them. I spoke to medical doctors and other health professional groups, news media personnel, and members of the general public. The questions were simple but required a fairly good understanding of HIV/AIDS to answer correctly. And the average score was low across the groups. More significantly, there were no significant differences among the three groups; that is, the doctors scored as low as the other groups (Duh, 1988).

Another important teacher of HIV/AIDS is non-governmental organizations or NGOs. Many of such organizations have sprung up in many African countries purposely to deal with the HIV/ AIDS epidemic. Many of them do an effective job in awareness creation, community mobilization, advocacy and stigma campaign. Local NGOs and other community-based organizations may be more effective than the media and government agencies in educating the public on HIV/AIDS because they are part of the communities and may be more trusted. However, many of them do not possess the requisite knowledge to do effective teaching and end up giving just facts. These NGOs should themselves acquire the necessary training for their staff so that they would be better able to teach the public.

To effect necessary behaviour change, education should not be limited to imparting understandable information on HIV/AIDS. Effort should be made to elicit personal behaviour information in order to provide the necessary advice. Here, health professionals can provide the best service both on individual and group bases. Doctors have been urged to take sexual and drug use history from their patients during routine clinic visits (Cates & Gowen, 1991). But there is evidence that many doctors are uncomfortable about sex and do not inquire about their patients' sexual practices, and even fewer doctors discuss HIV/AIDS with their patients on a regular basis (Gerbert, et al, 1990). Doctors in developing countries are even less likely to talk about sexuality during routine visits because of the fact that they tend to have too many patients during average clinic hours. They usually take minimal history relevant to the issue at hand in order to see as many patients as possible.

Health care professionals, the news media, and families have a recognized role in educating their respective clients on health matters. Each group plays a unique role and is guided by certain standards. Health care professionals and members of the news media provide health information based on the level of knowledge they possess on a particular topic and how comfortable they are with the issue. The news media are further restrained in what they can say or print based on certain legal and ethical principles. Families, at least in principle, can discuss any health topic in any detail they want. However, they are often constrained by certain traditional mores and do not discuss certain so-called taboo topics. With the arrival of HIV/AIDS, health education has been extended beyond the traditional health educators. People who may not be adequately trained, including some health care professionals, are asked to discuss sexual matters and do it explicitly.

The HIV/AIDS epidemic has created instant educators and counselors. Their job is to educate others on the disease and ways of preventing the spread of the epidemic. Some of them became HIV/AIDS educators by necessity because of their profession, example being doctors and other health care professionals. Others became educators either by choice or by society's expectations. The latter group includes churches, schools, parents, the news media, and famous personalities, so-called celebrities. Some of these educators have not accepted their new role well. For example, many doctors do not like discussing frank sexual matters with their patients either because they are uncomfortable about the issue or they believe they are not trained well enough for it. These doctors see their role as healers, and what people do in their bedrooms is a private matter. Also, medical specialization often makes it difficult for some doctors to discuss HIV/AIDS with their patients; demand of the specialty simply does not allow enough time to adequately study and understand the issue well.

Perhaps the most controversial issue about AIDS education is the role schools should play. Many teachers feel unqualified or uncomfortable to discuss HIV/AIDS and sexual or drug use matters. Furthermore, some segments of society do not believe the school is the place to discuss such matters. At issue are the questions of how early in school children should hear about those things and whether the discussion of safer involvement in certain activities could actually promote, instead of prevent, those activities. Yet schools are encouraged, and in some cases mandated, to provide sex education. The purpose of sex education, of course, is to prevent unintended pregnancies in addition to HIV/AIDS and other STIs. Is it the schools' responsibility to teach about pregnancy and STI prevention? What is the likely consequence of such education? At what grade level should explicit sexual matters be discussed?

Proponents of school-based sex education maintain that only explicit discussion is likely to yield the desired results. Students should understand the basics of human sexuality and be instructed on how to prevent transmission of HIV and other STIs, and pregnancy. They further assert that sex education should be started at the earliest age possible, certainly before young people become sexually active. Consequently, the school is the natural setting for sex education. Opponents counter that the consequence of explicit sex education may be more detrimental than good. The frank discussion of sex might lead young people to think about engaging in sexual intercourse when they might otherwise not think about it. And the discussion of safer sex methods would make them feel at ease and actually engage in sexual intercourse.

Dr. Karen Hein, who was the director of the adolescent AIDS program at Montefiore Hospital in New York, has stated that it is insufficient or even inappropriate to tell teenagers to be monogamous and know their partner. She was even more blunt

261

about her disagreement with abstinence: "....to try to stamp out sex among teenagers in America or any other country is tilting at windmills, an absurdity. Some of us seem not to want teenagers to learn about their own and others' bodies and, eventually, to enjoy intimacy." (Hein, 1993; p. 493).

Those who believe people should be free to have sex stress the need for "responsible sex"; that is, using condom for protection. And above all, they should be taught the proper way to use it and be advised to use it consistently. This has become the battle cry all over the world regarding HIV/AIDS prevention education.

What is a teenager to do then? The pressure to have sex may come from friends or even parents; and the media are saturated with messages of the glamour of sex. Pictures of half naked men and women are seen on television and in magazines. All kinds of products, from cars to beer, are advertised with sexual messages and suggestions. And some celebrities, whom young people may look up to, are referred to as sex symbols or heart throbs; some of them talk about sex as necessary and desirable. The popular American singer, Madonna, in promoting her new book which was simply entitled *Sex*, stated during a television interview: "The more people say sex is bad, the more I want to say no, it is not; no, it is not'." When asked about her reaction to the problem of unwanted pregnancy and deadly STIs, she said, "No risk, no glory."

HIV/AIDS education at the university level is, of course, less controversial since the students there are adults and choose to enrol in courses. But should such education be made mandatory at the universities? It is probably unnecessary or impractical to require university students to take a course on HIV/AIDS. However, making such courses available has proved useful in improving knowledge and changing attitudes about AIDS on some university campuses (Johnson et al, 1990; Strauss et al, 1992). In addition to teaching about HIV disease and prevention, such a course may involve discussions of how societies deal with contagion, stigma, disability, death, social stratification and access to scarce resources (Strauss et al, 1992).

Perhaps the most unconventional setting for HIV/AIDS education is the workplace. Since HIV/AIDS affects mostly people who are employed or are employable, employers have been forced to deal with HIV/AIDS in the workplace. It is in the interest of employers to educate their workers so as to prevent HIV infection in the work force. As stated in earlier chapters, many workers such as teachers, agricultural extension workers, and health care workers are dying in their numbers from HIV/AIDS in parts of Africa. In addition, workers have to be educated to alleviate their fears of working alongside co-workers who might have AIDS or HIV infection. For people employed by the health care system, there is the added need for education to overcome inhibitions about serving clients with HIV/AIDS. So, many companies offer workplace HIV/AIDS education to their employees, and some health care institutions require participation by all workers. Often employers invite experts from the outside to conduct the educational sessions, and some keep experts as regular consultants.

The question of whose job it is to educate about HIV/AIDS implicitly asks whose responsibility it is to pay for the educational programmes. Since the HIV/AIDS epidemic is of such mammoth proportions, it has been said that governments must be involved in its control. Indeed, the control of any illness that is a potential public health threat falls in the domain of the government. So when it comes to any type of formal HIV/AIDS education, the ultimate responsibility lies with the government. And governments at all levels—local, regional, and national—have been urged to take the leadership role in HIV/AIDS education. But many governments have not taken the leadership role, and they have been criticized for the lack of effective educational programmes (Duh, 1991; Des Jarlais et al, 1991).

In reality, all the educational programmes discussed in this chapter cannot be implemented without the direct or indirect involvement of the government. So, governments have mandated or instituted school-based HIV/AIDS education, work place HIV/AIDS education, and media campaigns. But the most important role of governments in this regard is the funding of the educational programmes, be it government-run or government supported. Thus governments at all levels have been called upon to invest in HIV/AIDS education. The response to this call has varied widely, but the overall response has not been adequate in proportion to the enormity of the pandemic.

The UNAIDS has been given (or has taken) the responsibility for the global control of HIV/AIDS, while national governments are supposed to be responsible for the control in their individual countries. So as the pandemic rages on and the need for education becomes clearer, UNAIDS and national governments have been urged to take the leadership role in educating the public about

HIV/AIDS. In many cases, when people say governments should take the leadership role in HIV/AIDS education, they really mean that the government should provide the needed funds for the education. This is exemplified by the fact that some HIV/AIDS workers expect or even ask for government financial involvement (assistance) but demand freedom from governmental involvement (interference) in the program content. This sometimes creates conflicts and controversy in some educational programs.

The responsibility of the government in educating the public on HIV/AIDS is rather broad since HIV/AIDS is a public health threat. Thus, not only does the government have responsibility for supportive role in governmental and non-governmental programs, some governments have done and are doing direct education through video materials, pamphlets, brochures, and public service announcements on radio and television. It is in this role of direct education that the governments can wield real power in influencing the content of educational material. These forms of relating information have the potential of reaching many people; therefore, the contents have to be accurate, up-to-date, understandable, and persuasive. In addition to these forms of direct involvement by governments, personal appearances and pronouncements on HIV/AIDS by heads of state or government can be very productive. The much touted and impressive reduction in HIV/AIDS prevalence rates in Uganda has been attributed to the very direct involvement of the president of that country in educating the Ugandan public. He has taken every opportunity to talk about HIV/AIDS, and that approach has yielded impressive results that need to be emulated elsewhere. Other heads of state and government should emulate the example set by the president of Uganda.

Conclusion

The answer to the question posed by the title of this chapter is at once simple and complex. Whose job is it to educate on AIDS? The simple answer is *everybody*. At the basic level, individuals can and should educate themselves and each other as health care personnel, as members of formal associations such as churches and civic groups, as members of the community, as members of the family, and as patients (of HIV disease). The answer is complex in that everybody may not be able or willing to educate. Lack of adequate knowledge or the uncomfortable feeling about discussing certain issues may be constraints. So the pragmatic response is that everybody should be *involved* in HIV/AIDS education. Those in a position to should teach and, more importantly, be allowed to teach, and the rest of us should be willing to learn from the "teachers".

The teachers of HIV/AIDS education should be schools, families, churches, the work place, doctors and other health care professionals, the news media, community-based organizations and the government. The education should be approached pragmatically, and all feasible means of effective education should be explored and employed. Thus, we should not permit arguments about taste and morality to interfere with the process. Likewise, the issue of turfdom should not be barriers to effective education. It has been said that doctors are the most knowledgeable about HIV/AIDS and thus the best teachers (Windom, 1988), but they should not have a monopoly over HIV/AIDS education. Furthermore, many doctors do not possess enough knowledge on the topic either because of their medical specialty or lack of interest in the issue. And in most cases, there are simply not enough doctors available to provide the varied services needed to control the HIV/AIDS epidemic. The important thing is that all the teachers should be themselves fully educated on their respective aspects of the issue so they can deal effectively with those aspects of the educational process.

The ultimate aim of HIV/AIDS education is to alley unfounded fears and to effect behaviour modification. To arrive at either endpoint, it is necessary to know where people are in terms of knowledge, beliefs and attitudes, and in terms of behaviours and practices. To this end, research is a necessary component of the educational process. Research is also necessary for the evaluation of programs. Thus, HIV/AIDS education necessarily requires some form of division of labour. For example, doctors and other health care professionals may teach about the biology of HIV/AIDS and conduct the necessary research; families and churches may teach about abstinence; news media personnel may teach about faithfulness to partners and condom use, and about new developments. By the same token, governments, non-governmental organizations, and businesses could be responsible for paying for the educational programs in addition to providing some education.

Division of labour obviously does not mean groups should not work together. Not only is it desirable but it is necessary that cooperation exist if fruitful outcome is to be achieved. Who does what, and how much groups or individuals do depend upon the community and available resources. For example, in some developing countries, the majority of the people get their information on HIV/AIDS through the news media. In such situations, members of the media should be well educated and provided with the latest information on HIV/AIDS.

Doctors and other HIV/AIDS educators may get their messages across through the media. People of celebrity status, such as soccer players and musicians in Africa, should be encouraged to be involved in HIV/AIDS education since they are often emulated by young people. As stated by the American actor, Rod Steiger, before a U.S. Senate committee: "For some strange reason, if you're a half-ass celebrity, people listen to what you say." Celebrities who accept the challenge and responsibility should be well informed on the particular issue of HIV/AIDS they intend to tackle.

Ultimately, the job of HIV/AIDS education rests with individuals. We should all try to educate ourselves and to take personal responsibility for our behaviour. In my speeches on HIV/AIDS, especially when I speak to students and other young people, I end the speeches by urging the members of the audience to go out and educate people in their neighbourhoods, schools, churches, families, workplaces, and everywhere the opportunity arises because HIV/AIDS education is everyone's business.

As stated earlier in this chapter, the question of whose job it is to educate the public implies whose job it is to pay for the education. Indeed the question applies to paying for the implementation of the comprehensive program because perhaps the biggest problem most governments in Africa are faced with in this regard is financial resources. Whether for the training of personnel, the building of facilities, the purchase of medicines and other supplies, or prevention programmes, money is the determining factor. It is indeed a tall order to ask for such a comprehensive approach to one disease when many of these governments are saddled with billions of dollars in foreign debt; some of them use as much as 50% of government budget allocations to service these debts. They have to use their meagre resources for other sectors of the health care system, education, agriculture, transportation, and several other government services. Furthermore, some of them are engaged in civil and territorial wars that are putting added strain on the already stretched economy. But HIV/AIDS is not just one disease; it is an epidemic with the potential to decimate whole populations in some countries, and it affects all the other government programs listed above. It is indeed a developmental problem.

The HIV/AIDS epidemic in Africa is so massive that it must be controlled and controlled comprehensively, whether the individual countries have the resources or not. The UNAIDS has estimated that it would require about 2 to 3 billion US dollars a year for education and prevention services in Africa. Obviously, a lot more would be needed for a comprehensive program of control and prevention. The UN Secretary General, Kofi Annan, announced the formation of a fund for the control of the HIV/AIDS pandemic and other major infectious diseases in developing countries at an international HIV/AIDS conference on Africa in Abuja, Nigeria, in April 2001. He estimated that 7 to 10 billion

US dollars would be needed for the fund and called on the international community to contribute to the fund. Former US president, Bill Clinton, stated during that conference that the international community could raise that amount quite easily. He added that, as far as his country was concerned, it was a matter of willingness, not ability, to come up with the money.

As stated by President Clinton, there is money available in the international community to help the poor countries combat the HIV/AIDS epidemic. The question is, are those with the money willing to give away the needed funds? The world's seven most industrialized countries plus Russia, the so-called G8 nations, promised in 1999 to write off $100 billion of poor country debt. This was partly to help them deal the HIV/AIDS epidemic, but by the end the year 2000, very little of those monies had been delivered (Oxfam, 2000). The United States, with an estimated 800,000 people living HIV/AIDS, had a budget of $7.7 billion for HIV/AIDS control for fiscal year 2001; that amount would be increased to $10 billion for fiscal 2002. For the same period of time, the U. S. government allocated $365 million, not even half a billion, for HIV/AIDS control in *all* developing countries where 95% of the world's 36. 1 million sufferers lived.

Mr. Annan did initiate the Global Fund for HIV/AIDS, Tuberculosis, and Malaria, with headquarters in Geneva, Switzerland, in 2002. The purpose of the Global Fund is to provide financial resources for governments and organizations in resource poor countries to combat these three infectious diseases whose combined effects are truly devastating to poor countries. Rich countries, big companies and even wealthy individuals are supposed to make contributions to the Fund in the range of 7-10 billion dollars. Mr. Annan made a personal contribution of US$100,000 to the Fund at its inception. Contributions to the Fund have not been as expected, and the Global Fund has not accumulated anywhere near the 7-10 billion dollars it needs.

Between 2001 and 2005, contributions to the Global Fund came from more than 50 countries, foundations, corporations, and private individuals. During that period, the Fund acquired US$2.5 billion for HIV/AIDS programming, much less than needed in Africa. Indeed some officials of the Global Fund expressed the fear that the Fund might run out money if donations did not pick up substantially. Meanwhile, several countries in Africa have been able to acquire significant amounts of money from the Global Fund and other sources to implement programmes, especially in relation to the provision of ARV.

In addition to the Global Fund, a major boost to some African countries has been the US President's Emergency Plan for HIV/AIDS Relief (PEPFAR). Started in 2003, the PEPFAR was a five-year initiative worth US$15 billion. This initiative was for only 15 focus countries—Botswana, Cote d'Ivoire, Ethiopia, Guyana, Haiti, Kenya, Mozambique, Namibia, Nigeria, Rwanda, South Africa, Tanzania, Uganda, Vietnam, and Zambia. The PEPFAR had a strong emphasis on treatment and care, with 70% going for treatment and palliative care (55% and 15% respectively), and 20% and 10% respectively going for prevention and orphans and vulnerable children programmes.

In this state of affairs, I believe individual governments in Africa should develop their respective sound and workable strategic plans to combat the epidemic in their respective countries. They should readjust their national budgets to make substantial amounts available for HIV/AIDS control. Indeed, the 2001 Abuja Declaration called for African governments to allocate 15% of their national budgets to health in order to adequately fight the three diseases. Then they should raise the rest of the funds from other sources within and outside the country. They should build alliances by contacting private businesses, NGOs, foundations, and governments of rich nations. In this regard, multilateral agencies such as the World Bank World Bank, United States Agency for International Development (USAID), the British Department for International Development (DfID), the Japanese International Cooperation Agency (JICA), and the Danish International Development Agency (DANIDA) have been quite helpful to some Africa countries.

African countries should build and strengthen close working relationship with these international agencies in their fight against the HIV/AIDS epidemic. There should be mechanisms built into their strategic plans for monitoring and evaluation of programmes in order to assure donors and their own people that the monies are used efficiently. In other words, the programmes should be results oriented. By building alliances with the groups listed above, there should be partnerships with the entities so that aid would not just be in the form of financial assistance but also other in kind assistance.

REFERENCES

1. American Health Consultants (1993). Studies on male sexual behaviour: safe sex not an accepted practice. *AIDS Alert* 8; 88-90
2. Cates, W. & Gowen, G.S. (1991). HIV infection: primary care counseling and testing needed more than ever. *Modern Medicine* 59; 65-72.
3. Des Jarlais, D.C. & Stephenson, B. (1991). History, ethics, and politics in AIDS prevention research, *American Journal of Public Health*, 81,1393-1394.
4. Duh, S.V. (1988). Educating the public on AIDS: how much do the educators know? Presented at the IV International Conference on AIDS, Stockholm, June 1988. Abstract#6036.
5. Duh, S.V. (1991). *Blacks and AIDS: Causes and Origins*; Newbury Park: Sage Publications.
6. Fineberg, H.V. (1988). The social dimensions of AIDS. *Scientific American* 259; 128-134.
7. Gerbert, B., Maguire, B.T., Coats, T.J. (1990). Are physicians talking to their patients about AIDS? *American Journal of Public Health* 90; 511-1513.
8. Global Fund (2006). Monthly progress update —15 November 2005. Available at *www.theglobalfund.org.* Accesses25/106
9. Hein, K. (1993). "Getting real" about HIV in adolescents. *American Journal of Public Health* 83; 492-494.
10. Johnson, J.A., et al (1990). Knowledge and attitudes about AIDS among first- and second-year medical students. *AIDS Education and Prevention* 2, 48-57
11. Strauss, R.P., et al (1993). Cognitive and attitudinal impacts of a university AIDS course: interdisciplinary education as a public health intervention. *American Journal of Public Health* 83, 569 572.
12. Windom, R.E. (1988). "We are your sons, your daughters..." *Public Health Reports* 103; 209 210
13. Youth Research Working Paper (2006). Impact of sexual and HIV education programs on sexual behaviors of youth in developing countries. *YouthNet,* 1-4